# HEALTH CAREER PLANNING

# HEALTH CAREER PLANNING
*A Realistic Guide*

## Ellen Lederman, M.S.

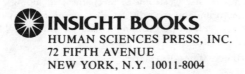

**INSIGHT BOOKS**
HUMAN SCIENCES PRESS, INC.
72 FIFTH AVENUE
NEW YORK, N.Y. 10011-8004

*For Andy*

**Library of Congress Cataloging-in-Publication Data**

Lederman, Ellen F.
  Health career planning.

  Bibliography: p.
  Includes index.
  1. Allied health personnel—Vocational guidance.
2. Career development.  I. Title.  [DNLM: 1. Allied
Health Personnel.  2. Career Choice.  3. Health
Occupations. W 21.5 L473h]
R697.A4L425     1987      610.69'53'023      87-21391
ISBN 0-89885-397-4 (hard)
        0-89885-401-6 (paper)

Copyright © 1988 by Human Sciences Press, Inc.
72 Fifth Avenue, New York, New York 10011
An Insight Book

Printed in the United States of America
987654321

# CONTENTS

# INTRODUCTION

I thought I knew what I was getting into when I went into occupational therapy, but it's turned out to be a lot different than I thought it would be. I never dreamed that it would be such exhausting work. I thought I'd go home every night feeling very upbeat and good about myself, but I've found that half the time I leave feeling incredibly tired and discouraged. It's hard to always feel *up* when you're working with sick people. Progress is often very slow and sometimes you never see any at all.

When I was a student, I had this vision of myself as a miracle worker, being able to help every patient assigned to me. But now I've been forced to come to terms with the fact that I can't help everyone—and that some patients don't want my help, and a few don't even want to get better! I thought I'd be appreciated and liked by all my patients, but in reality, that hasn't been the case. I realize now that a lot of the patients aren't in a position to recognize and appreciate my efforts; they're too busy dealing with their own problems.

Sometimes my self-esteem gets pretty low. When I can't help a patient as much as I'd like, I feel powerless and ineffectual. It doesn't help that most of the physicians have been slow to recognize the value of OT and to really treat us like we're members of the team. And there are times when I feel bad because my salary is so much lower than my college friends who majored in business and other areas.

Even so, I still don't regret becoming an occupational therapist, but I wish I had had a more realistic idea of what it would be like. If I had known exactly what to expect from the beginning, I would have been better prepared to deal with the realities of a health care career.

—Occupational therapist,
Albuquerque, New Mexico

Surprises are part of most areas of life, but when it comes to your career, you want to make it as sure a thing as possible. When you choose your lifework, you want to make certain you understand what it really involves. Insufficient knowledge and idealized expectations can be disastrous. You'll only be disappointed, frustrated, or even angry when you eventually discover that the realities of your career are far different from what you had anticipated.

If you're thinking about entering a health career, you particularly need to be sure that you know what to expect. While you cannot fully understand every aspect of a job before you actually experience it, you should familiarize yourself as much as possible with all its various duties and demands. Even if you're positive that a certain career is right for you, be sure to read all of Chapter 1.

There are over 200 different health careers, some of which you might never have heard of, but which might better utilize your skills and provide more satisfaction than the field you were originally considering. It's not enough simply to want a health career; you need to find the one that comes closest to filling your needs as well as making the most of your talents.

Anyone who is planning to pursue a health career also needs to read Chapter 2 to prepare for the challenges that lie ahead as a health care student. If you're already enrolled in a health curriculum, this chapter can help you understand and cope with the special stresses of studying for a health career.

Students and new health care professionals will find that Chapter 3 addresses one of the hardest stages in a health career:

the first year or two. Making the transition from the college campus to the work world is not easy. You're expected to function as a full-fledged health care worker, but you lack the experience and confidence to really feel comfortable in your new role. This chapter takes up the problems typical of this period and offers practical suggestions on how to deal with them.

Workers in the middle years of their careers will want to focus on Chapter 4. This chapter recognizes the fact that even experienced health care professionals can have unresolved problems and conflicts in this stage of their careers. There are important decisions to make about what direction your career should be taking; Chapter 4 will help you develop the strategies you need.

If you've been involved in a health career for many years, Chapter 5 should be of special interest. This chapter discusses how you can maximize your remaining years of work. These last years can and should be more than just marking time until retirement. You do need to start planning for your retirement, but you also need to make sure that your last work years are productive and fulfilling.

Workers at any stage of their careers should read Chapter 6. Health care is a highly demanding field that can tax your physical and psychological reserves. In most health care jobs, employees aren't sitting at a desk shuffling papers. They're lifting patients, carrying heavy equipment, and reaching and bending 8 or more hours each day. The emotional demands can be equally draining. Any job in which you deal with people can be stressful; this stress is intensified when you deal with people who are in pain, discomfort, or emotional turmoil. It is unrealistic to believe that the physical and emotional demands can ever be eliminated entirely. But with the help of Chapter 6, you can learn how to meet the stresses of a health career and avoid burnout.

There may come a point in your career when you feel that you no longer want to remain in health care. Chapter 7 can help you make the switch into a different field. The decision to leave a health career is a major one, so you need to fully understand your motives and needs when contemplating such a move. The chapter also offers strategies for making the move once you know for sure that a health career is no longer right for you.

Health careers can be arduous and frustrating, but they can

also be challenging and rewarding. Whatever career stage you're currently in or whatever your particular field may be, *Health Career Planning: A Realistic Guide* provides a starting point for understanding the problems of a health career and for developing mechanisms for coping with them. Make a commitment to doing everything you can to make the most of your health career; you'll find that your time and efforts were well spent.

*Ellen Lederman*

*Chapter 1*

# DECIDING ON A HEALTH CAREER

Health care seemed like the logical career choice for me since I wanted to work with people. I couldn't see myself looking at a computer all day long or worrying about sales figures every month. Although both my parents are successful businesspeople, I knew that I wouldn't be happy in the business world. I definitely wanted a helping profession.

Deciding that I wanted a career in health care was easy. The hard part came when I tried to narrow it down to a specific field. I didn't really know anything about any of the allied health careers; nursing was the only field I was vaguely familiar with, but I didn't think I wanted to be a nurse. My high school guidance counselor wasn't much help. She gave me a booklet on health careers and left me on my own to decide. Flipping through the book, I happened to notice the paragraph on dietitians. A career in dietetics seemed like it could have possibilities. While it was definitely a helping profession that would allow me to work with sick people, it wouldn't require me to perform any procedures that would make me squeamish, like injecting people or cleaning

wounds. Best of all, it involved food and I certainly have
had a lifelong interest in that!

But once I was enrolled in a dietetics program in college,
I began to suspect that it might not be the right career for
me. I hadn't realized how much biochemistry was involved.
Unfortunately, chemistry has never been my best area.
Somehow, though, I made it through school and became a
registered dietitian.

After a few years of working as an R.D., I still have
doubts about my career. I went into this field to work with
people, but I haven't had much patient contact in a long
time. My responsibilities now are mostly administrative and
I can't say I'm enjoying it a whole lot. Managing the dietary
department isn't much different than running any other
business. I have to worry about budgeting, ordering supplies,
and supervising employees. I'm not sure I want to be doing
this for the next 30 years. I can see now that I should have
put more thought into choosing my career.

—Dietitian,
Hartford, Connecticut

A career in nursing or allied health doesn't begin on your
first day on the job, nor on the day you graduate from school.
It actually begins on the day you decide you want to pursue a
health career. It's a decision that will affect the rest of your life,
so it's vital to really think it through.

## GENERAL CAREER CONSIDERATIONS

Your career decision will ultimately affect many other areas
of your life. One of the most obvious consequences of your choice
will be your financial situation. Since all of us who are not independently wealthy have to rely on our salaries for both the
necessities and luxuries of life, the career paths we choose have
a lot to do with our life-styles. High-paying fields enable a higher
standard of living. People who dream of big homes, sports cars,
cruises, and designer clothes need a career that holds the possibility of high enough pay to afford such things. Those for whom

glamorous living is not as important have a wider variety of career options, since they are not restricted to just those fields that may offer big money.

Career decisions affect life-styles in other ways besides finances. A person's job will determine the amount of free time he has. Many of the fields that offer status and high pay require much more than a 40-hour week. Whether the overtime is spent at the office or working home, people in such positions have less leisure than workers in other fields. For some people, this need not be a consideration because they derive a major portion of their personal satisfaction from work. But for others, work is mainly a way to pay the bills. Leisure time is of utmost concern to those with strong avocational interests.

Even social life is affected by the career choice. Adults tend to get to know people through their work. When contemplating a career option, reflect on the type of people who seem to gravitate toward that field. If they do not seem appealing as social companions, consider why a particular personality type goes into the field and why you would tend not to want to form personal friendships with them. Do their values seem different from yours? Do they seem too competitive and high-strung? Do they seem overly intellectual, or perhaps not as intelligent and cultured as you prefer? If you feel that you wouldn't want to socialize with them, that they're not on your wavelength, chances are you would be out of your element working with them, too.

In addition to providing a paycheck, jobs also allow us to express our personalities and talents. We all have certain personal traits and abilities that we bring to our work. Unfortunately, all too often, those characteristics don't match the requirements and demands of the job. Extroverts who work well with others may find themselves in a position that doesn't offer much interpersonal contact. Creative people may wind up in a structured, routine job that doesn't ask for ideas and innovative thinking. Since we usually spend 8 hours a day at work, the consequences of being in the wrong job are pervasive. There's nothing worse than constantly facing a workday that you find endlessly boring, stressful, or void of personal satisfaction.

There is no foolproof method for choosing the right career, but you'll be well on your way if you take the time for some probing self-analysis. Determine what's important to you. Most of all, be totally honest with yourself. This is not the time to fantasize or depict yourself as the kind of person whom you'd love to be. Viewing yourself in an idealized image, with the qualities you *want* to cultivate, may boost your self-esteem, but it will steer you wrong in making an appropriate decision. But don't just concede your weaknesses. Also assess your strong points. What do people praise about you? Don't be falsely modest. Admit to yourself what you excel in, what special abilities you can bring to a job.

## A SHORT SELF-QUIZ

There are more comprehensive personal inventories offered in career books or at career counseling or psychologists' offices, but this will get you started. There are no right or wrong answers. Only *you* know which ones best describe who you are and what you want from a job.

A). *What You Can Offer a Job*
Out of the following characteristics and talents, which one do you feel you're strongest in? Which one is your weakest area?
_____ Ability to work well with other people.
_____ Ability to solve problems.
_____ Mechanical ability.
_____ Ability to follow directions.
_____ Ability to work independently.
_____ Analytical ability.
_____ Creativity.
_____ Manual dexterity.
_____ Physical stamina and strength.
_____ Attention to details.
_____ Scientific aptitude.
_____ Other _____
_____

B). *What a Job Can Offer You*
Which of the following characteristics and rewards would you most like to receive from your job? Which is least important to you?

_____ High pay.

_____ Responsibility.

_____ Opportunity to help other people.

_____ Opportunity to be creative.

_____ Opportunity to solve problems.

_____ Prestige.

_____ Intellectual stimulation.

_____ Security.

_____ Comfortable working conditions.

_____ Opportunity to see your efforts result in a finished product.

_____ Limited stress.

_____ Other _____

_____

The next step is to explore the various career fields. Again, you need to do this as realistically and as honestly as possible. Don't fall for the television image of the medical field. Naturally, the interest here is in the high drama that has story value, not in the grueling day-to-day routine. As the hero of the life-and-death drama, the physician is dedicated and devoted, caring and compassionate, always making the right decisions, chivalrous to the nurses, with plenty of time for everybody. Seldom until the *St. Elsewhere* show were doctors portrayed as human beings with their own idiosyncracies.

Forget the fast-paced scenes on your TV screen of glistening hospital corridors, delivery, surgery, and private patient rooms, where the crisis culminates in triumph for the medical team. Think about the actual routine duties associated with the job rather than the aura of suspense, magical knowledge, and hairbreadth survival, which are the tools of the scriptwriters, not of the health care staff.

Qualities that stir you when you see them dramatically personified, no job can instill in you unless you possess these innate characteristics. You may long to see yourself as part of an inspired, healing community, but the job isn't going to impart to you any gift or power that is not potential within you.

## SPECIFIC CONSIDERATIONS FOR HEALTH CAREERS

Health care, rapidly becoming the largest industry in this country, offers such a diversity of career fields that there is virtually one to suit almost any individual's characteristics, abilities, and interests. There are over 200 different health careers, each with unique demands, responsibilities, and rewards. Some health careers may be right for you; whereas others will not.

Too many well-meaning people decide that they want a health career because they want to "*help* others" or "work with *people*." Many occupations, both in and out of the health field, will allow you to work with people. Being a counselor, teacher, or librarian is as much a helping occupation as those in the health field. It could be that a different "helping profession" would be more ideally suited for you than one of the more obvious health career choices.

There is no generic health career. There are only specific health careers, each with its unique duties, demands, work environment, educational and personal requirements, and rewards. Don't think your career dilemma is solved once you decide that you want to go into health care. Only when you know *exactly* which health career you want will you have chosen a career for yourself.

The following pages realistically pinpoint the personal qualifications, educational/training requirements, work environments and demands, and rewards associated with the various health occupations. The scope of this book does not permit detailed descriptions of each field; the reader who needs this information can refer to one of the books that deal exclusively with this subject arca. While some health occupations may have been left out of the following analysis (as based in part on *200 Ways to Put Your Talent to Work in the Health Field*© 1985, National Health Council,

Inc., New York City), it will introduce you to most of the major fields. The descriptions are all self-explanatory. Exact salary figures are not given since they can vary significantly from one year to the next or between different locales. Therefore, salaries are described as low (the bottom third of all nursing/allied health salaries), middle (middle third), and high (top third). Data for physicians, dentists, podiatrists, chiropractors, and optometrists are not included since these are not considered allied health personnel.

## HEALTH OCCUPATIONS DIRECTORY

### Clinical Laboratory Services

*Clinical Chemists*—perform complex chemical tests and procedures to analyze body tissues and fluids.

*Personal qualifications:*

Aptitude for physics, biology, and (especially) chemistry.

Orientation to detail.

Ability to follow procedures exactly as designated.

Ability to work independently.

*Educational/training requirements:*

Master's degree in chemistry (Ph.D. preferred).

*Work environment and demands:*

Hospitals or clinical laboratory settings.

Sedentary; long standing or sitting in one spot.

Minimal patient contact.

Work may involve unpleasant odors.

May have to handle dangerous/toxic substances (but if handled carefully, minimal danger is involved.

*Rewards:*

Salaries generally fall within high-middle to high range for allied health personnel.

Satisfaction of helping to detect disease so that it can be properly diagnosed and treated.

*Contact:*

American Association for Clinical Chemistry
1725 "K" St., NW
Suite 1010
Washington, D.C. 20006

*Cytotechnologists*—screen slides of human cells to detect cancer.

*Personal qualifications:*

Aptitude for biological sciences.

Orientation to detail.

Ability to work independently.

Good visual functioning.

*Educational/training requirements:*

2 years of college, followed by 1-year program at a school of cytotechnology.

*Work environment and demands:*

Hospitals or clinical laboratory settings.

Sedentary; long standing or sitting in one spot.

Work may be the same from day to day.

*Rewards:*

Salaries generally fall within low to middle range for allied health personnel.

Satisfaction of helping to detect disease so that it can be properly diagnosed and treated.

*Contact:*

American Society of Cytology
130 S. 9th St.
Philadelphia, PA 19107

*Histologic technicians*—cut, stain, and mount body tissues for microscopic examination by pathologists.

*Personal qualifications:*

Orientation to detail.

Ability to perform procedures exactly as designated.

Moderate manual dexterity.

*Educational/training requirements:*

1-year training program at hospitals and laboratories.

*Work environment and demands:*

Hospitals or clinical laboratory settings.

Minimal patient contact.

Sedentary; long standing or sitting in one spot.

Work may seldom vary from day to day.

May have to handle dangerous/toxic substances (but, if handled carefully, there is minimal danger involved).

*Rewards:*

Salaries generally fall within the low range for allied health personnel.

Satisfaction of helping physicians to diagnose and treat disease.

*Contact:*

American Society of Clinical Pathologists
2100 W. Harrison St.
Chicago, IL 60612

*Medical laboratory technicians*—carry out medical laboratory tests under the direction of medical technologists.

*Personal qualifications:*

Aptitude for biological, chemical, and physical sciences.

Orientation to details.

Ability to follow procedures exactly as designated.

Ability to work under minimal supervision.

*Educational/training requirements:*

2-year associate degree in medical laboratory technology.

*Work environment and demands:*

Hospitals or clinical laboratories.

May have minimal patient client.

Sedentary; long standing or sitting in one spot.

Work may seldom vary from day to day.

May have to handle dangerous/toxic substances (but, if handled correctly, there is minimal danger involved).

*Rewards:*

Salaries generally fall within the low range for allied health personnel.

Satisfaction of helping to detect disease so it can be properly diagnosed and treated.

*Contact:*

International Society for Clinical Laboratory Technology
818 Olive Street
Suite 918
St. Louis, MO 63101

*Medical technologists*—perform complex tests to determine the presence or absence of disease.

*Personal qualifications:*

Aptitude for biological, physical, and chemical sciences.

Orientation for details.

Ability to follow procedures exactly as designated.

Ability to work independently.

Supervisory abilities.

*Educational/training requirements:*

3 years of college with concentration in the sciences, plus 1 year at a hospital school of medical technology.

*Work environment and demands:*

Hospitals or clinical laboratories.

May have minimal patient contact.

Sedentary; long standing or sitting in one place.

Work may seldom vary from day to day.

May need to supervise technicians and assistants.

May have to handle dangerous/toxic substances (but, if handled carefully, there is minimal danger involved).

*Rewards:*

Salaries generally fall within the middle range for allied health personnel.

Satisfaction of helping to detect disease so that it can be properly diagnosed and treated.

*Contact:*

American Society for Medical Technology
330 Meadow Fern Drive
Suite 200
Houston, TX 77067

*Microbiologists*—perform laboratory tests in the field of microbiology.

*Personal qualifications:*

Aptitude for physical, chemical, and especially, biological sciences.

Orientation to detail.

Ability to follow designated procedures.

Good visual functioning.

Ability to work independently.

*Educational/training requirements:*

At least a 4-year bachelor's degree in a science plus 1 year of lab experience.

*Work environment and demands:*

Hospitals or clinical laboratories.

Sedentary, involving long standing or sitting in one spot.

May specialize in a particular area and work may seldom vary from day to day.

Work may involve unpleasant odors.

*Rewards:*

Salaries generally fall within middle range for allied health personnel.

Satisfaction of helping to detect disease so that it can be properly diagnosed and treated.

*Contact:*

American Society for Microbiology
1913 Eye St., NW
Washington, DC 20037

*Dentistry*

*Dental assistants*—maintain supplies, schedule appointments, keep records, process X rays, prepare patients for examination, and assist the dentist at chairside.

*Personal qualifications:*

Ability to relate well to others.

Ability to follow procedures exactly as directed.

Moderate manual dexterity.

*Educational/training requirements:*

Certificate, diploma, or associate degree from 1- or 2-year program at a community college or vocational-technical program.

*Work environment and demands:*

Dental offices.

A combination of office duties and patient contact.

Amount of pressure depends on the dentist's practice.

*Rewards:*

Salaries generally fall within low to middle range for allied health personnel.

Satisfaction of helping dentist treat oral diseases and disorders.

*Contact:*

American Dental Assistants Association
666 N. Lake Shore Drive
Suite 1130
Chicago, IL 60611

*Dental hygienists*—examine, clean, and polish teeth, take X rays, give fluoride treatments, and educate patients about caring for their teeth and gums.

*Personal qualifications:*

Moderate aptitude for biological sciences.

Good manual dexterity.

Orientation to detail.

Ability to work independently, with minimal supervision from dentist.

Ability to motivate others to strive towards dental health.

*Educational/training requirements:*

2 year associate degree from a community college or 4 year college degree.

*Work environment and demands:*

Dental offices.

Intensive patient contact.

Amount of pressure depends on the dentist's practice.

*Rewards:*

Salaries generally fall within the middle range for allied health personnel, but may sometimes be in the high range if the hygienist is paid incentives and bonuses for treating large number of patients.

Satisfaction of promoting dental health.

*Contact:*

American Dental Hygienists Association
444 N. Michigan Ave.
Chicago, IL 60611


*Dental technicians*—make and repair dentures, crowns, and bridges.

*Personal qualifications:*

Artistic ability.

Orientation to detail.

Good vision.

High degree of manual dexterity.

Tendency to be a perfectionist.

Ability to work with minimal supervision, but according to dentist's prescriptions.

*Educational/training requirements:*

2-year certificate or associate degree programs at community colleges.

*Work environment and demands:*

Dental laboratories.

Minimal patient contact.

May be under pressure to process large amounts of work quickly while still maintaining quality.

Fairly sedentary; long sitting.

*Rewards:*

Salaries generally fall within middle range for allied health personnel.

Satisfaction of seeing tangible results of one's work and of providing quality products for dentists to utilize.

*Contact:*

National Association of Dental Laboratories
3801 Mount Vernon Ave.
Alexandria, VA 22305

## Dietetics

*Dietitians*—utilize nutrition to promote health, prevent and treat illness. Duties may include instruction on proper diets, planning of menus and special diets, and management of food services.

*Personal qualifications:*

Aptitude for biology and chemistry.

Orientation to detail.

Ability to relate well to others.

Ability to work independently.

Teaching ability.

Ability to motivate others towards good nutrition.

Management/supervisory skills (if in charge of a food service department).

Creative ability (to plan unique menus and diets).

*Educational/training requirements:*

4-year college degree plus a dietetic internship.

*Work environment and demands:*

Hospitals, nursing homes, clinics, private practice, community settings.

May involve supervisory/administrative duties (ordering supplies, budgeting, supervising food service workers) in addition to patient contact.

*Rewards:*

Salaries generally fall within the middle range for allied health personnel, but may reach high levels for supervisory positions or private practices.

Satisfaction of helping others become healthier through proper diet.

*Contact:*

American Dietetic Association
430 N. Michigan Ave.
Chicago, IL 60611

*Dietetic technicians and dietetic assistants*—assist dietitians in planning menus and supervising food production.

*Personal qualifications:*

Moderate aptitude for biological and chemical sciences.

Orientation to detail.

Ability to relate well to others.

Ability to be creative while following established guidelines.

Ability to work under the supervision of dietitians.

*Educational/training requirements:*

1 year program at community colleges or vocational-technical schools for dietetic assistants;

2 year associate degree for dietetic technicians.

*Work environment and demands:*

Hospitals, nursing homes, community settings.

*Rewards:*

Salaries generally fall within low range for allied health personnel.

Satisfaction of assisting dietitian's efforts in helping others to become more healthy through a proper diet.

*Contact:*

American Dietetic Association
430 N. Michigan Ave.
Chicago, IL 60611

## Education

*Public health educators*—educate the public and consult with other health personnel about disease and how to prevent it.

*Personal qualifications:*

Aptitude for biological, chemical, psychological, and social sciences.

Analytical abilities.

Teaching ability.

Ability to relate well to others.

Creativity for program planning.

Ability to work independently.

*Educational/training requirements:*

Master's degree in public health or community health education.

*Work environment and demands:*

Hospitals and community agencies.

May involve consultative work, necessitating travel.

*Rewards:*

Salaries generally fall within middle to high ranges for allied health personnel.

Satisfaction of promoting health on individual and community levels.

*Contact:*

Society for Public Health Educators
703 Market Street
Suite 535
San Francisco, CA 94103

*School health educators*—teach elementary, secondary, and college students about health.

*Personal qualifications:*

Teaching ability.

Aptitude for biological and psychosocial sciences.

Ability to relate well to others, particularly young people.

Creativity for program planning.

Ability to work independently.

*Educational/training requirements:*

4-year college degree in health education.

*Work environment and demands:*

Elementary or secondary schools or colleges.

If employed in public schools, may involve other, non-health education duties (i.e., being a cafeteria monitor or bus supervisor).

May involve a 9-month work schedule with a 3-month long summer vacation.

*Rewards:*

Salaries fall within middle range for allied health personnel.

Satisfaction of teaching children, adolescents, and young adults about maintaining and promoting their health.

*Contact:*

American School Health Association
1521 S. Water Street
Box 708
Kent, OH 44240

*Specialists for the visually handicapped*—work with visually impaired children and adults. Orientation and mobility instructors teach clients how to travel independently indoors and outdoors. Rehabilitation teachers teach daily living skills such as braille communication, hygiene, cooking, and recreation. Teachers of the visually handicapped teach special communication skills or assist with regular studies.

*Personal qualifications:*

Teaching ability.

Patience.

Ability to relate well to others.

Ability to work independently.

Problem-solving abilities.

Creativity in planning individualized instruction.

Ability to motivate others.

*Educational/training requirements:*

Bachelor's degree in education or rehabilitation.

*Work environment and demands:*

Community centers for the blind, rehabilitation centers, public and private schools.

Intensive student/client contact.

*Rewards:*

Salaries generally fall within low (i.e., in nonprofit centers for the blind) to middle range (i.e., public school system) for allied health personnel.

Satisfaction of helping visually impaired children and adults to lead independent lives.

*Contact:*

American Foundation for the Blind
15 W. 16th St.
New York, NY 10011


## Health Information and Communication

*Health sciences librarians*—provide medical and health-related information to health professionals. Duties include locating reference information, choosing and purchasing books and journals, organizing information, and administering the library.

*Personal qualifications:*

Good reading skills.

Ability to work independently.

Ability to organize items.

Teaching abilities (to instruct students and professionals in use of resources).

Analytical ability.

Administrative skills (i.e., planning, budgeting).

Interest in media (print, film, videotape).

*Educational/training requirements:*

Master's degree in library science with courses in health sciences librarianship.

*Work environment and demands:*

Medical/health professional schools, hospital libraries, libraries in medical or health-related businesses.

Work can range from fairly sedentary tasks (i.e., cataloging) to active tasks (i.e., reaching and bending to retrieve books and films).

Some work is solitary, but generally involves moderate contact with health professionals.

*Rewards:*

Salaries generally fall within the middle range for allied health personnel.

Satisfaction of helping health professionals improve their knowledge and skills by providing them with pertinent information.

*Contact:*

Medical Library Association
919 N. Michigan Ave.
Chicago, IL 60611

*Medical illustrators*—create graphics for publications, film, television, exhibits, and three-dimensional modules.

*Personal qualifications:*

Strong artistic abilities (drawing, painting, sculpting, commercial art).

Aptitude for anatomy and general medical knowledge.

Ability to work independently.

Orientation to detail.

Tendency to be a perfectionist.

*Educational/training requirements:*

Training in certified schools with art, anatomy, and medical sciences; though employment possible as a graphic artist from a noncertified school.

*Work environment and demands:*

Medical schools, research centers, book publishers, television or film production.

Mostly sedentary.

Work can be solitary or in cooperation with medical researchers, writers, and teachers.

*Rewards:*

Salaries generally fall within middle range for allied health personnel, but may reach the high range if self-employed or in certain media jobs.

Satisfaction of contributing to medical and health information through artistic efforts, as well as seeing very tangible results of one's work.

*Contact:*

Association of Medical Illustrators
2692 Huguenot Springs Road
Midlothian, VA 23113


*Medical records administrators*—prepare and analyze statistical reports, design patient information systems, and supervise records department.

*Personal qualifications:*

Computer aptitude.

Orientation to detail.

Aptitude for statistics.

Good reading skills.

Analytical skills.

Supervisory skills.

Basic understanding of medical science and terminology.

*Educational/training requirements:*

4-year bachelor's degree in medical records administration

or a 1-year certificate program after achieving a bachelor's degree in another area.

*Work environment and demands:*

Hospitals, clinics, nursing homes, other health facilities.

Long sitting.

May entail supervisory duties.

*Rewards:*

Salaries generally fall within middle range for allied health personnel.

Satisfaction of making sure that complete, accurate records are kept, thus ensuring that patients receive appropriate care from medical providers.

*Contact:*

American Medical Record Association
875 N. Michigan Ave.
Chicago, IL 60611

*Medical records technicians*—check records for completeness, index medical information, and help medical records administrators prepare reports.

*Personal qualifications:*

Computer aptitude.

Orientation to detail.

Good reading skills.

Basic understanding of medical terminology.

*Educational/training requirements:*

2-year associate degree.

*Work environment and demands:*

Hospitals, clinics, nursing homes.

Long sitting.

Mostly solitary work.

*Rewards:*

Salaries generally fall within low to middle range for allied health personnel.

Satisfaction of helping to maintain complete, accurate records, thus ensuring that patients receive appropriate care from medical providers.

*Contact:*

American Medical Record Association
875 N. Michigan Ave.
Chicago, IL 60611

*Medical transcriptionists*—type and prepare dictated medical reports.

*Personal qualifications:*

Typing/word processing/computer skills.

Good spelling and grammar.

Basic understanding of medical terminology.

*Educational/training requirements:*

No formal training; may be trained on the job.

*Work environment and demands:*

Hospitals, other health facilities, large medical practices.

Long sitting.

Mostly solitary work; possible interaction with physicians and other health personnel.

May be under some pressure to produce reports quickly.

*Rewards:*

Salaries generally fall within the low range for allied health personnel.

Satisfaction of helping to maintain complete, accurate records, thus ensuring that patients receive appropriate care from medical providers.

*Contact:*

American Medical Record Association
875 N. Michigan Ave.
Chicago, IL 60611

*Medical/science/technical writers*—write or edit health information for the public and for professionals.

*Personal qualifications:*

Excellent writing skills.

Good research skills.

Ability to work independently.

Understanding of basic and medical sciences and terminology.

*Educational/training requirements:*

Usually a college degree in journalism or English, supplemented by science courses.

*Work environment and demands:*

Newspapers, magazines, radio, television, professional journals, universities, foundations, government agencies, or free-lance writing of books and articles.

*Rewards:*

Salaries generally fall within middle range for allied health personnel, although some self-employed writers may achieve incomes in the high range.

Satisfaction of helping to dissemimate health information to the public and to professionals, as well as seeing tangible results of one's work.

*Contact:*

National Association of Science Writers
P.O. Box 294
Greenlawn, NY 11740


## Health Services Administration

*Health service administrators*—assume management roles in health-related institutions, organizations, and programs.

*Personal qualifications:*

Leadership ability.

Financial management skills.

Analytical skills.

Problem-solving skills and decision-making ability.

Personnel management skills.

*Educational/training requirements:*

Master's degree in hospital administration, public health,

or public administration, although some positions only require a 4-year bachelor's degree in these fields.

*Work environment and demands:*

Hospitals, nursing homes, clinics, other health-related institutions, health associations, government regulatory agencies.

Long sitting.

May continually be under intense pressure to work within budget, balance the books, and solve complex problems.

Limited patient contact, but frequent interaction with department heads and other personnel.

*Rewards:*

Salaries generally within the high range for allied health personnel.

Satisfaction of making decisions and setting policies that ultimately affect the delivery of health care.

*Contact:*

American College of Health Care Administrators
8120 Woodmont Ave., Suite 200
Bethesda, MD 20814

## Medicine

*Emergency medical technicians*—provide immediate care to critically ill or injured people while transporting them to emergency rooms at a medical center.

*Personal qualifications:*

Aptitude for biology and chemistry.

Ability to understand medicine and medical terminology.

Ability to work under stress and pressure.

Ability to relate well to people.

Moderate manual dexterity.

Ability to apply book knowledge to practical situations.

Ability to work independently.

*Educational/training requirements:*

81-hour course approved by the U.S. Department of

Transportation. EMT-Dispatcher rating requires additional training. Courses are given by community colleges, hospitals, and fire, health, and police departments.

*Work environment and demands:*

Ambulance or rescue services.

Physical demands of lifting patients and administering cardiac resucitation.

Intense emotional stress of dealing with patients and their families in emergency situations.

*Rewards:*

Salaries generally fall within middle range for allied health personnel.

Satisfaction of providing first-line care and even saving patients' lives.

*Contact:*

National Association of Emergency Medical Technicians
P.O. Box 627
Boulder, MT 59632

*Medical assistants*—assist doctors by performing clinical and clerical duties, such as typing, billing, scheduling appointments, preparing patients for examinations, and performing simple laboratory tests.

*Personal qualifications:*

Basic understanding of medical terminology.

Clerical skills (i.e., typing, bookkeeping).

Ability to interact effectively with patients, physicians, and other personnel.

Ability to take direction from the physician.

*Educational/training requirements:*

1-year certificate or 2-year associate degree programs at vocational-technical schools and community colleges.

*Work environment and demands:*

Physicians' offices.

Actual demands vary according to the physician's practice,

but will usually involve a combination of clerical and clinical duties.

*Rewards:*

Salaries generally fall within the low to middle range for allied health personnel.

Satisfaction of helping physicians run their practices, thus contributing indirectly to the health of the patients.

*Contact:*

American Association of Medical Assistants
20 N. Wacker Dr.
Chicago, IL 60606

*Physician assistants/associates*—perform routine patient care tasks under the direction of a physician, including examinations, treatments, prescribing certain drugs, and educating patients.

*Personal qualifications:*

Aptitude for biology and chemistry.

Excellent understanding of medicine.

Ability to effectively interact with a wide variety of patients.

Ability to work independently, as well as to accept direction from the physician.

Moderate manual dexterity.

Ability to apply book knowledge to practical situations.

*Educational/training requirements:*

Usually 2 years of college with a concentration in the sciences, followed by a 2-year training program (at colleges, medical schools, or in the military) leading to a certificate, associate, or bachelor's degree.

Prior health care experience may substitute for some college.

*Work environment and demands:*

Hospitals, clinics, physician's offices.

Intensive patient contact.

Varied responsibilities, depending on the work situation.

Can be physically demanding (i.e., lifting patients) and emotionally stressful.

*Rewards:*

Salaries generally fall within middle to upper range for allied health personnel.

Satisfaction of providing direct medical care to patients, promoting their health and treating their illnesses.

*Contact:*

Association of Physician Assistant Programs
1117 N. 19th St.
Arlington, VA 22209

## Nursing

*Licensed practical nurses*—promote physical, mental, and social well-being of patients.

*Personal qualifications:*

Excellent interpersonal skills.

Aptitude for biomedical science.

Moderate manual dexterity.

Good physical stamina.

Ability to follow procedures as directed.

*Educational/training requirements:*

1-year training program at a school of practical nursing.

*Work environment and demands:*

Hospitals, nursing homes, physicians' offices, home health agencies.

Physically and emotionally demanding.

*Rewards:*

Salaries generally fall within low to middle range for allied health personnel.

Satisfaction of promoting health in a variety of patients.

*Contact:*

National Federation of Licensed Practical Nurses
P.O. Box 11038
214 S. Driver St.
Durham, NC 27703

*Registered nurses*—promote physical, mental, and social well-being of patients.

*Personal qualifications:*

Excellent interpersonal skills.

Strong aptitude for biological, chemical, physical, and psychological sciences.

Moderate manual dexterity.

Good physical stamina.

Ability to carry out prescribed protocols as well as exercise independent judgment.

*Educational/training requirements:*

2-year associate degree; 3-year hospital diploma; or 4-year bachelor's degree.

*Work environment and demands:*

Hospitals, nursing homes, schools, clinics, physicians' offices, businesses, home health agencies.

Physically and emotionally demanding.

*Rewards:*

Salaries generally fall within the middle range for allied health personnel.

Satisfaction of promoting health in a variety of patients.

*Contact:*

National League for Nursing
10 Columbus Circle
New York, NY 10019

## Pharmacy

*Pharmacists*—prepare and fill prescription drugs.

*Personal qualifications:*

Excellent aptitude for biomedical sciences.
Orientation to details.

*Educational/training requirements:*

5-year college program.

*Work environment and demands:*

Hospitals, clinics, drug stores.

May involve long standing.

*Rewards:*

Salaries generally fall within middle to high ranges for allied health personnel.

Satisfaction of contributing to other people's health through the proper dispensing of pharmaceuticals.

*Contact:*

American Association of Colleges of Pharmacy
4720 Montgomery Lane, Suite 202
Bethesda, MD 20814

## Physical and Psychosocial Rehabilitation

*Art therapists*—utilize art media to effect positive change in the emotional status of children and adults.

*Personal qualifications:*

Excellent interpersonal skills.

Artistic talent.

Creativity.

Aptitude for psychological and social sciences.

Analytical abilities.

*Educational/training requirements:*

Master's degree in art therapy.

*Work environment and demands:*

Psychiatric facilities, schools for the emotionally disturbed, nursing homes.

Emotionally, rather than physically, demanding work.

*Rewards:*

Salaries generally fall within the middle range for allied health personnel.

Satisfaction of helping to improve the emotional well-being of other people.

*Contact:*

American Art Therapy Association

1980 Isaac Newton Square, S.
Reston, VA 22090

*Athletic trainers*—prevent and rehabilitate athletic injuries, following prescription of the team physician. Duties include health education, first aid, and purchasing and fitting athletic equipment.

*Personal qualifications:*

Aptitude for anatomy and physiology.

Good interpersonal skills.

Moderate manual dexterity.

Ability to work independently in carrying out physician's orders.

Physical strength and stamina.

Ability to think and react quickly.

*Educational/training requirements:*

Graduate degree in athletic training preferred.

College graduates without an athletic training degree can qualify by completing additional courses and a minimum of 1800 hours supervised clinical experience.

*Work environment and demands:*

On the playing field, training camps, locker rooms.

Can be physically challenging at times—i.e., lifting, supporting players.

*Rewards:*

Salaries generally fall within the middle to upper ranges, depending on the type of athletic team.

Satisfaction of promoting and restoring health of athletes.

*Contact:*

National Athletic Trainers Association
1001 E. Fourth St.
Greenville, NC 27834

*Dance therapists*—utilize dance to effect positive change in the emotional or physical status of children and adults.

*Personal qualifications:*

Excellent interpersonal skills.

Dancing talent.

Creativity.

Aptitude for psychological, social, and biological (i.e., kinesiology) sciences.

Good physical stamina.

*Educational/training requirements:*

Master's degree in dance therapy.

*Work environment and demands:*

Psychiatric facilities, rehabilitation centers, nursing homes, schools for the physically handicapped or emotionally disturbed.

Can be emotionally demanding.

Very physically active.

*Rewards:*

Salaries generally fall within the middle range for allied health personnel.

Satisfaction of helping to improve the emotional or physical well-being of other people.

*Contact:*

American Dance Therapy Association
2000 Century Plaza, Suite 108
Columbia, MD 21044

*Music therapists*—utilize music to effect positive change in the emotional status of children and adults.

*Personal qualifications:*

Excellent interpersonal skills.

Musical talent.

Creativity.

Aptitude for psychological and social sciences.

*Educational/training requirements:*

At least a bachelor's degree in music therapy; master's degree preferred.

*Work environment and demands:*

Psychiatric facilities, rehabilitation centers, nursing homes, special education settings.

Moderate physical activity.

*Rewards:*

Salaries generally fall within the middle range for allied health personnel.

Satisfaction of helping to improve the emotional or physical well-being of other people.

*Contact:*

American Association of Music Therapy
66 Morris Ave.
P.O. Box 359
Springfield, NJ 07081

*Occupational therapists*—utilize purposeful activity and adaptive equipment to help children and adults lead independent and satisfying lives.
May work with people who are mentally, emotionally, or physically handicapped.

*Personal qualifications:*

Excellent interpersonal skills.

Aptitude for biological and psychological sciences.

Creativity.

Moderate manual dexterity.

Adequate physical stamina.

Ability to instruct and motivate others.

*Educational/training requirements:*

Bachelor's degree in occupational therapy. College graduates with degrees in other areas can train through a 2-year master's degree program.

*Work environment and demands:*

Hospitals, psychiatric facilities, nursing homes, schools, clinics, home health agencies.

Can be emotionally and physically demanding.

*Rewards:*

Salaries generally fall within the middle range for allied health personnel.

Satisfaction of helping all types of people learn or regain the skills that are necessary for living a productive life.

*Contact:*

American Occupational Therapy Association
1383 Piccard Drive
Rockville, MD 20850


*Occupational therapy assistants*—utilize purposeful activity and adaptive equipment (under the direction of an occupational therapist) to help children and adults lead independent and satisfying lives.

May work with people who are emotionally, mentally, or physically handicapped.

*Personal qualifications:*

Excellent interpersonal skills.

Aptitude for biological and psychological sciences.

Creativity.

Moderate manual dexterity.

Adequate physical stamina.

Ability to instruct and motivate others.

*Educational/training requirements:*

2-year associate degree.

*Work environment and demands:*

Hospitals, psychiatric facilities, nursing homes, schools, clinics.

Can be physically and emotionally demanding.

*Rewards:*

Salaries generally within the lower to middle range for allied health personnel.

Satisfaction of helping all types of people learn or regain the skills necessary for living a productive life.

*Contact:*

American Occupational Therapy Association
1383 Piccard Drive
Rockville, MD 20850

*Orthotists and prosthetists*—fabricate and fit artificial limbs (prosthetists) or orthopedic splints and braces (orthotists). Can work in either or both areas.

*Personal qualifications:*

Aptitude for anatomy.

Orientation to detail.

Excellent manual dexterity.

Good interpersonal skills.

Tendency to be a perfectionist when constructing projects.

*Educational/training requirements:*

Bachelor's degree in orthotics or prosthetics, plus 1 year of clinical experienced.

(May be other alternatives for those with associate or bachelor's degrees in other areas, such as 2 years of clinical experience and taking specialized courses).

*Work environment and demands:*

Hospitals, rehabilitation centers, physician's offices, clinics.

*Rewards:*

Salaries generally fall within middle to upper ranges for allied health personnel.

Satisfaction of efforts resulting in a finished product that will enable disabled people to lead independent lives.

*Contact:*

American Board for Certification in Orthotics and Prosthetics
717 Pendleton St.
Alexandria, VA 22314

*Physical therapists*—utilize exercise, heat, cold, water, or electricity to restore physical function of children and adults.

*Personal qualifications:*

Strong aptitude for biological, physical, and psychosocial sciences.

Excellent interpersonal skills.

Excellent physical stamina.

Ability to instruct and motivate others.

Ability to work independently.

*Educational/training requirements:*

4-year degree in physical therapy. College graduates with degrees in other areas can take a 1- or 2-year program leading to a certificate or a master's degree.

*Work environment and demands:*

Hospitals, rehabilitation centers, clinics, physicians' offices, schools, home health agencies.

Physically and emotionally demanding.

*Rewards:*

Salaries generally within the middle range for allied health personnel if employed in a hospital. Therapists employed in a physician's office, home health agency on a contract basis, or private practice may earn salaries in the upper range.

Satisfaction of restoring physical function, independence, and relieving pain.

*Contact:*

American Physical Therapy Association
1111 N. Fairfax St.
Alexandria, VA 22314

*Physical therapy assistants*—under the direction of a physical therapist, utilize exercise, heat, cold, water, or electricity to restore physical function of disabled children and adults.

*Personal qualifications:*

Good aptitude for biological, physical, and psychosocial sciences.

Excellent interpersonal skills.

Excellent physical stamina.

Ability to instruct and motivate others.

Ability to follow designated procedures.

*Educational/training requirements:*

2-year associate degree in physical therapy assisting.

*Work environment and demands:*

Hospitals, rehabilitation centers, clinics, physicians' offices, schools.

Physically and emotionally demanding.

*Rewards:*

Salaries generally fall within middle range for allied health personnel.

Satisfaction of restoring physical function, independence, and relieving pain.

*Contact:*

American Physical Therapy Association
1111 N. Fairfax St.
Alexandria, VA 22314

*Psychiatric/mental health technicians*—work with mentally ill patients under the supervision of nurses, physicians, or other personnel. Duties include observation, basic interviewing, and counseling of patients, as well as helping them with their daily treatment, self-care, and recreation programs.

*Personal qualifications:*

Excellent interpersonal skills.

*Educational/training requirements:*

Requirements vary according to employer. A 2-year associate degree in psychology, social or human services is usually appropriate.

*Work environment and demands:*

Psychiatric hospitals; community programs.

*Rewards:*

Salaries generally fall within the low range for allied health personnel.

Satisfaction of helping patients to improve their mental health and lead productive lives.

*Contact:*

American Health Care Association
1200 15th St.
Washington, DC 20005

*Psychologists*—investigate and apply knowledge about human behavior to mental health problems.

*Personal qualifications:*

Excellent aptitude for psychology.

Excellent interpersonal skills.

Strong analytical skills.

Creativity.

*Educational/training requirements:*

At least a 2-year master's degree in psychology.

Many positions require a doctoral degree.

*Work environment and demands:*

Hospitals, rehabilitation centers, clinics, schools, work settings, community programs.

Can be emotionally demanding.

*Rewards:*

Salaries generally within middle to upper range for allied health personnel.

Satisfaction of helping to solve behavioral problems and promoting mental health.

*Contact:*

American Psychological Association
1200 17th St., NW
Washington, D.C. 20037

*Rehabilitation counselors*—help physically or emotionally disabled persons obtain and adjust to a job.

*Personal qualifications:*

Excellent interpersonal skills.

*Educational/training requirements:*

2-year master's degree program in rehabilitation counseling.

*Work environment and demands:*

Rehabilitation hospitals, community programs.

*Rewards:*

Salaries generally within the middle range for allied health personnel.

Satisfaction of helping people realize their full potential in life, including holding a satisfying job.

*Contact:*

National Rehabilitation Counseling Association
633 S. Washington St.
Alexandria, VA 22314

*Social workers*—help individuals, groups, and communities find solutions to problems (i.e., relating to employment, housing, finances).

*Personal qualifications:*

Excellent interpersonal skills.

Aptitude for psychological and social sciences.

Creativity and problem-solving skills.

*Educational/training requirements:*

A master's degree is required for most positions, although some jobs only require a bachelor's degree in social work.

*Work environment and demands:*

Hospitals, psychiatric and rehabilitation facilities, nursing homes, clinics, home health agencies, community settings.

Can be emotionally demanding.

*Rewards:*

Salaries generally within the middle range for allied health personnel.

Satisfaction of helping people to solve their problems and promote change within the community.

*Contact:*

National Association of Social Workers

7981 Eastern Ave.
Silver Spring, MD 20910

*Speech-language pathologists and audiologists*—evaluate and treat speech and language problems (speech-language pathologists) or hearing disorders (audiologists). Some clinicians specialize in both areas.

*Personal qualifications:*

Excellent interpersonal skills.

Aptitude for biological and psychological sciences.

Ability to instruct and motivate others.

*Educational/training requirements:*

Master's degree in speech-language pathology and/or audiology.

*Work environment and demands:*

Hospitals, rehabilitation facilities, nursing homes, schools, home health agencies, clinics, private practices.

Can be emotionally draining.

*Rewards:*

Salaries generally within the middle range for allied health personnel, although some speech pathologists/audiologists in private practices may earn more.

Satisfaction of helping children and adults learn or relearn to communicate and to make the most of their hearing.

*Contact:*

American Speech-Language-Hearing Association
10801 Rockville Pike
Rockville, MD 20852

*Therapeutic recreation specialists*—utilize recreational activities to help disabled children and adults maximize their leisure time satisfaction.

*Personal qualifications:*

Excellent interpersonal skills.

Good physical stamina.

Creativity.

Ability to instruct and motivate others to participate in recreation.

*Educational/training requirements:*

Minimum of a bachelor's degree in recreation or therapeutic recreation; master's degree preferred.

*Work environment and demands:*

Hospitals, rehabilitation centers, nursing homes, residential schools, community agencies and centers.

Can be physically active.

*Rewards:*

Salaries generally within the middle range for allied health personnel.

Satisfaction of helping people to enjoy their leisure time.

*Contact:*

National Therapeutic Recreation Society
3101 Park Center Drive
Alexandria, VA 22302

## Podiatry

*Podiatric assistants*—assist podiatrists in patient care (including surgical assisting and plaster casting) and office management.

*Personal qualifications:*

Excellent interpersonal skills.

Good manual dexterity.

Ability to follow directions and perform procedures as designated.

Office skills.

*Educational/training requirements:*

1-year certificate or 2-year associate degree program.

*Work environment and demands:*

Podistrists' offices.

*Rewards:*

Salaries generally fall within the low to middle ranges for allied health personnel.

Satisfaction of helping to promote and improve foot health.

*Contact:*

American Podiatric Medical Association
20 Chevy Chase Circle, N.W.
Washington, D.C. 20015

## Science and Engineering

*Biomedical engineers*—utilize engineering methods to solve biological and medical problems such as designing equipment for diagnostic and therapeutic purposes.

*Personal qualifications:*

Excellent aptitude for biology, physics, and mathematics.

Analytical and problem-solving skills.

*Educational/training requirements:*

At least a 4-year bachelor's degree in engineering or physics. Some positions may require a master's degree in biomedical engineering.

*Work environment and demands:*

Hospitals, rehabilitation centers, research facilities, businesses.

*Rewards:*

Salaries generally within the middle to high ranges for allied health personnel.

Satisfaction of solving crucial medical problems and seeing efforts culminate in a finished product.

*Contact:*

Alliance for Engineering in Medicine and Biology
1101 Connecticut Ave., N.W.
Suite 700
Washington, D.C. 20036

*Biostatisticians*—help solve basic research problems related to health care by using mathematics and statistics.

*Personal qualifications:*

Excellent mathematical aptitude.

Analytical skills.

Interest in research.

*Educational/training requirements:*

A minimum of a bachelor's degree with a major in statistics. Full professional status necessitates training at the master's level.

*Work environment and demands:*

Hospitals, universities, community agencies, research centers.

*Rewards:*

Salaries generally fall within the middle to high ranges for allied health personnel.

Satisfaction of helping to solve crucial health-related problems.

*Contact:*

American Statistical Association
806 15th St., N.W.
Suite 640
Washington, D.C. 20005

## Technical Instrumentation

*Electroencephalographic (EEG) technologists and technicians*—operate the EEG machine which records electrical brain activity.

*Personal qualifications:*

Excellent interpersonal skills.

Ability to follow procedures exactly as designated.

*Educational/training requirements:*

6 months training for technicians; 1 year for technologists. While some community colleges offer associate degree programs for technologists, it is possible for technicians to train on the job or in formal training programs at hospitals and clinics.

*Work environment and demands:*

Hospitals and clinics.

*Rewards:*

Salaries generally fall within the low range for allied health personnel.

Satisfaction of helping physicians to diagnose brain disorders.

*Contact:*

American Society of Electroencephalographic Technologists
6th at Quint
Carroll, Iowa 51401

*Nuclear medicine technologists*—use radioactive materials to diagnose and treat disease.

*Personal qualifications:*

Good interpersonal skills.

Aptitude for biological, chemical, and physical sciences.

Ability to follow procedures exactly as designated.

Orientation to detail.

*Educational/training requirements:*

Generally a 1- or 2-year program at a community college, university, or hospital. Some college coursework in the sciences may be required prior to admission.

*Work environment and demands:*

Hospitals, clinics, doctors' offices.

Work requires the handling of radioactive materials, so extreme caution must be consistently practiced.

*Rewards:*

Salaries generally fall within the middle range for allied health personnel.

Satisfaction of helping physicians diagnose and treat disease.

*Contact:*

Society of Nuclear Medicine
136 Madison Ave.
New York, NY 10016

*Radiation therapy technologists/X-ray technicians*—utilize X rays or other radiation for diagnostic or therapeutic purposes.

*Personal qualifications:*

Excellent interpersonal skills.

Aptitude for physics and biology.

Orientation to details.

Ability to follow designated procedures.

Some mechanical aptitude for handling machines.

*Educational/training requirements:*

Generally a 2-year program at hospitals or community colleges. Some colleges offer 4-year bachelor's degrees.

*Work environment and demands:*

Hospitals, clinics, physicians' offices, mobile X-ray services.

Safety procedures must be consistently followed to minimize worker's exposure to radiation.

*Rewards:*

Salaries generally fall within the low to middle ranges for allied health personnel.

Satisfaction of performing a service that enables physicians to diagnose and treat illness.

*Contact:*

American Society of Radiologic Technologists
15000 Central Ave., S.E.
Albuquerque, N.M. 87123

*Respiratory technicians*—administer oxygen, gases, or aerosol drugs to patients with cardiopulmonary dysfunction.

*Personal qualifications:*

Excellent interpersonal skills.

Good aptitude for biological, physical, and chemical sciences.

Some mechanical aptitude for dealing with machines.

Orientation to details.

Ability to follow designated procedures.

*Educational/training requirements:*

1-year program at a hospital.

*Work environment and demands:*

Hospitals, clinics, physicians' offices, mobile respiratory services.

Work can be emotionally stressful due to the critical nature of the services and the acute illnesses of the patients.

*Rewards:*

Salaries generally fall within the low to middle ranges for allied health personnel.

Satisfaction of improving the cardiopulmonary health of patients.

*Contact:*

American Association for Respiratory Therapy
1720 Regal Row
Dallas, TX 75235

*Respiratory therapists*—administer oxygen, gases, or aerosol drugs to patients with cardiopulmonary dysfunction. They may also perform diagnostic testing relating to respiratory function.

*Personal qualifications:*

Excellent interpersonal skills.

Excellent aptitude for biological, physical, and chemical sciences.

Some mechanical aptitude for dealing with machines.

Orientation to detail.

Ability to follow designated procedures.

*Educational/training requirements:*

2-year associate or 4-year bachelor's degree.

*Work environment and demands:*

Hospitals, clinics, physicians' offices, mobile respiratory services.

Can be emotionally stressful due to the critical nature of the services and the acute illnesses of the patients.

*Rewards:*

Salaries generally within the middle range for allied health personnel.

Satisfaction of improving the cardiopulmonary health of patients.

*Contact:*

American Association for Respiratory Therapy
1720 Regal Row
Dallas, TX 75235

*Surgical technologists* (operating room technicians)—prepare the operating room and patients for surgery, as well as handling surgical instruments to the surgeon during an operation.

*Personal qualifications:*

Good interpersonal skills.

Ability to follow designated procedures.

Orientation to detail.

*Educational/training requirements:*

9- to 12-month certificate or 2-year associate degree programs.

*Work environment and demands:*

Operating rooms in hospitals and outpatient surgical facilities.

May require long standing.

*Rewards:*

Salaries generally within the middle range for allied health personnel.

Satisfaction of facilitating surgical procedures for surgeons, thus contributing indirectly to patients' health.

*Contact:*

Association of Surgical Technologists
8307 Shaffer Parkway
Littleton, CO 80127

## Veterinary Medicine

*Animal technicians*—assist veterinarians in the handling and care of animals. Duties may include feeding, dressing wounds, collecting specimens, performing simple lab tests, assisting with medical and surgical procedures, and keeping records.

*Personal qualifications:*

Interest in animals and the ability to relate well to them, as well as to their owners.

Some aptitude for biological sciences.

Orientation to detail.

Ability to follow designated procedures.

Physical strength.

*Educational/training requirements:*

Generally a 2-year associate degree.

*Work environment and demands:*

Veterinary offices and hospitals, zoos.

Can be physically demanding work (i.e., lifting heavy animals).

*Rewards:*

Salaries generally fall within the low ranges for allied health personnel.

Satisfaction of working with and contributing to the health of animals and to the peace of mind of pet owners.

*Contact:*

American Veterinary Medical Association
930 N. Meacham Road
Schaumberg, IL 60196


## Vision Care

*Dispensing opticians*—make and fit eyeglasses or lenses prescribed by opthalmologists and optometrists.

*Personal qualifications:*

Good interpersonal skills.

Excellent aptitude for physics.

Orientation to detail.

Ability to perform procedures exactly as designated.

Good manual dexterity.

*Educational/training requirements:*

2-year associate degree or four years of on-the-job training in an apprenticeship program.

*Work environment and demands:*

Optometrists' offices, optical stores.

*Rewards:*

Salaries generally fall within the middle to upper ranges for allied health personnel.

Satisfaction of seeing efforts result in a finished product that will improve people's vision.

*Contact:*

Opticians Association of America
10341 Democracy Lane
Fairfax, VA 22030


*Ophthalmic assistants*—perform simple vision testing, obtain patient histories, change eye dressings, and administer oral medications.

*Personal qualifications:*

Excellent interpersonal skills.

Ability to perform procedures exactly as designated.

*Educational/training requirements:*

1-year training program.

*Work environment and demands:*

Ophthalmologists' offices.

*Rewards:*

Salaries generally fall within the low range for allied health personnel.

Satisfaction of assisting ophthalmologists with eye care.

*Contact:*

Joint Commission on Allied Health Personnel in Ophthalmology
1812 N. St. Paul Rd.
St. Paul, MN 55109

*Ophthalmic technicians*—assist the ophthalmologist surgery, make optical measurements, and perform other technical skills.

*Personal qualifications:*

Excellent interpersonal skills.

Orientation to detail.

Aptitude for biology and physics.

Ability to perform procedures as designated.

*Educational/training requirements:*

2-year associate degree.

*Work environment and demands:*

Ophthalmologists' offices.

*Rewards:*

Salaries generally fall within the low to middle range for allied health personnel.

Satisfaction of assisting ophthalmologists with eye care.

*Contact:*

Joint Commission on Allied Health Personnel in Ophthalmology

1812 N. St. Paul Rd.

St. Paul, MN 55109

*Optometric assistants*—assist optometrists by performing office and simple patient duties, such as helping patients with frame selection and ordering prescribed lenses.

*Personal qualifications:*

Good interpersonal skills.

Ability to perform office work.

*Educational/training requirements:*

1-year certificate or diploma program.

*Work environment and demands:*

Optometrists' offices.

*Rewards:*

Salaries generally fall within the low range for allied health personnel.

Satisfaction of directly contributing to the eye care and appearance of a variety of patients.

*Contact:*

American Optometric Association
243 N. Lindbergh Blvd.
St. Louis, MO 63141

*Optometric technicians*—assist optometrists in skilled patient activities like vision training and testing.

*Personal qualifications:*

Excellent interpersonal skills.

Good aptitude for physics and biology.

Orientation to details.

Ability to perform procedures as designated.

*Educational/training requirements:*

2-year associate degree in paraoptometrics.

*Work environment and demands:*

Salaries generally fall within the low to middle ranges for allied health personnel.

Satisfaction of promoting optometric health by helping to test and train vision.

*Contact:*

American Optometric Association
243 N. Lindbergh Blvd.
St. Louis, MO 63141

*Orthoptists*—correct crossed eyes in children and adults by the use of special exercises.

*Personal qualifications:*

Excellent interpersonal skills.

Good aptitude for physics and biology.

Orientation to detail.

Ability to perform procedures as designated.

*Educational/training requirements:*

2-years of college followed by a 24-month training program in an eye clinic or hospital.

*Work environment and demands:*

Ophthalmologists' offices, eye clinics and hospitals.

*Rewards:*

Salaries generally fall within the middle ranges for allied health personnel.

Satisfaction of helping to correct vision problems.

*Contact:*

American Orthoptic Council
3914 Nakoma Road
Madison, WI 53711

### FURTHER POINTS IN ZEROING IN ON A HEALTH CAREER

Now that you've had a brief review of the majority of possible health careers, you should be better able to determine if one of them is right for you. On the basis of the answers from the self-quiz earlier in this chapter, see if you find a career that utilizes some of your strengths. If, for example, the self-quiz revealed that your strongest area is creativity, you might not be happy in a clinical laboratory career such as microbiology or cytotechnology in which you need to follow established procedures. If your strength is your interpersonal skills, you may want to avoid a career in a field like biostatistics or medical records in which your contact with patients and staff might be more limited than in, say, dental hygiene or physical therapy.

Likewise, be wary about choosing a career that requires a personal characteristic or talent that you've designated as your weakest area. While it is true that weaknesses can be compensated to some extent, it is usually best to avoid those fields in which the skills and characteristics that you're lacking are crucial. It's perfectly acceptable to want to be challenged, and to venture into new territory, but there is only so far that you can rise to a challenge before it becomes too frustrating and stressful. So if you know you're "all thumbs," don't choose a career such as dental technology or orthotics which require precision manual skills. Your dexterity would probably improve somewhat with practice, but why not utilize those skills you *do* have? Similarly, if computers faze you, you may not be comfortable in medical records. If you don't have a lot of stamina and strength, you are probably not up to physical therapy.

The educational/training requirements for the different allied health occupations generally range from 1-year certificate programs to 6 or more years of college and graduate studies. Long years of college study are not for everyone, so be careful that the health occupation you choose doesn't require more training time than you're willing and able to commit yourself to. Some people are limited to only a year or two of study at a community college since they can't afford more time or tuition. Others just don't relish the prospect of all those years of school. If 4 or more years of college aren't appealing, you won't be able to consider certain health careers, but you'll still have many options to choose from. But be sure you don't write off a college education too quickly for the wrong reasons. If the cost seems prohibitive, keep in mind that scholarships and loans are often available for health students. Before you decide that you couldn't possibly afford 4-plus years of schooling, speak with the department heads and financial aid officers of the colleges you would be interested in attending. They will be able to inform you of the availability of financial aid.

Don't automatically assume that you won't like college or won't do well because of your high school experience. Your record to date may *not* prove you're not a natural student. Quite often, people find that they really enjoy college and get far better grade point averages than they had in high school simply because they've become more mature and motivated. They're not so apt to daydream, and talk on the phone, and do all their work "the night before." This is especially true with health care students. Whereas certain high school courses may have seemed to have little to do with your life ("Give 5 causes of World War I"; "Name 2 dynamic characters in *Silas Marner*") health care courses are usually practical and relevant. Students who were just average performers in high school often blossom in college, particularly when they've made a commitment to a major that they intend to be their life's work, and can see where they are heading.

If you find yourself drawn to a particular health field but still aren't sure you want to commit yourself to all those years in school, remember that you don't necessarily have to attend school on a full-time basis. It may be possible to attend part-time or even to take off a year or two between degrees. For example, social work and speech pathology generally consider the master's degree to be the entry level for professional status, but that doesn't mean that you have to go to college for 4 years straight and then immediately go to graduate school. You can get your undergraduate degree first and work for a while before you return to school to get your graduate degree. You can also break up 4 years of college by first getting an associate degree in liberal arts or sciences and later returning to college to get your bachelor's in a health field.

The work *environment* is another key consideration in choosing a health care career. Some people are happiest in a setting with lots of other people and activity; the hospital environment can be ideal for this personality type. Other people feel more comfortable in a circumscribed, secluded, intimate, personalized environment. When deciding on a specific health care career, be sure that you could be happy in the typical work environments of that field. For example, if you dislike being closely confined within the same cubicle day in, day out, at the same desk or table, you may get cabin fever if your job plants you in a laboratory or doctor's office.

*Any* job, whether within or outside of the health care system, has *some* stress; but some health fields have unique characteristics which make that field especially demanding. Certain health jobs can be particularly stressful on a physical and/or emotional level. Some involve frequent lifting of patients or heavy machines. Others require long periods of standing. Jobs with heavy patient contact can take an emotional toll. It can be extremely taxing to work with people whose illnesses or disabilities are causing intense pain, anxiety, rage, fear, confusion, and disorientation. This is not to warn that these jobs be avoided; there are true satisfactions and rewards for workers in such fields. But if past experiences tend to suggest that your physical or emotional resources may not be sufficient to withstand the stressors of some health jobs, it may be wise to choose a job with less *built-in* stress.

We all base our career choices on the expectations of certain rewards. Some people choose a specific career because of the money. Others choose careers for less tangible fulfillment, such as opportunities to be creative or to have an impact on other people's lives. Make sure that the career you choose can offer the rewards that are most important to *you*. There are a few jobs that manage to combine high pay, prestige, intellectual stimulation, job security, full benefits, congenial coworkers, comfortable working conditions, and limited stress; but such jobs are few and far between. You can dream about such a job, but keep in mind that most of your peers have the same dream. Competition is fierce and the probability of your ever getting that dream job is quite remote, so you need to target a career that you can realistically pursue. Once you accept the fact that you can't find a job that offers *everything*, look for career fields that are likely to reward you with whatever comes first with you.

Health careers can be deeply rewarding, but usually in other than financial ways. Every health career offers the opportunity to help other people. Workers in some fields help in an indirect way (i.e., a biostatistician uses statistics to help solve health problems faced by communities, ethnic groups, and even entire countries). Most health workers directly contribute to the health and well-being of other people on a one-on-one basis. Some health careers would allow you to be creative, whereas others would provide you with the opportunity to use technical or scientific skills. Working in some health careers can reward you with the opportunity to see your efforts result in a finished product, providing tangible reinforcement. For example, an optician's efforts culminate in a pair of corrective eyeglasses that provide 20/20 vision and an orthotist sees his or her labor result in a splint or brace that will result in restored mobility. The majority of health fields, though, are more *process*-oriented than *result*-oriented. In many fields, workers do not have the gratification of a finished product at the end of the day. Quite often, they have *no* tangible means of *measuring* their effectiveness. If you have the need to see concrete results of your work on a consistent basis, you may not be happy in some of the therapy fields in which days and even weeks can go by before you know you've actually made a difference in a patient's life.

Many people are interested in finding work that rewards them with social status and prestige. There is nothing unworthy about seeking a career field that will offer that. But if prestige matters to you, chances are slim that you'll be happy in a nursing or allied health career. For various reasons, these fields have never been prestigious. In the hospital social structure, allied health workers usually find that they have second-class status. Physicians are clearly the ones with power and status; in addition to significantly higher pay and ultimate authority, they're even rewarded with plusher libraries and fancier dining rooms at the hospital. Outside of the hospital, health careers are also not held in high esteem by the general public. Society has become increasingly business-oriented, according its respect and admiration to successful businesspeople. Workers in health fields aren't part of the power or financial structure and consequently, their contributions to society frequently go unnoticed and unappreciated.

A corollary of low status is low pay. Health care workers typically aren't rewarded with salaries on a par with those of business and professional people. Some health fields offer higher salaries than others; but even these salaries can't begin to compete with the financial renumeration of most physicians, lawyers, accountants, and advertising executives. If you hope to make a lot of money, don't choose a nursing or allied health career. This is not to say that everyone who goes into a health career is committed to privation. On the contrary, many nursing and allied health workers manage to lead fulfilling lives on their salaries. Salaries for some health occupations are quite respectable, particularly in supervisory positions, private practices, or fields where there is a shortage of qualified personnel. Although there have not been any dramatic jumps in health care workers' salaries, they have been slowly but steadily increasing. Many analysts predict that salaries will significantly increase in an effort to entice more people to choose and remain in a health care career.

Until salaries increase substantially, health care workers have to live on the salaries they get. Even if your ultimate goal in life isn't just to earn as much as you possibly can, make sure that you'll be able to live on the anticipated salary of the health field you're interested in. Contact the professional association of that field to find out what its workers can expect to earn. Even more importantly, read the classified ads in the area where you plan to live so you can see exactly what salaries are offered in that locale.

Once you know what you'd be likely to earn in your chosen field, do a little bit of mathematical computations to see if you could live on that salary. You might decide that you can't consider a certain health career because you feel that you couldn't on less than $30,000, but you also might discover that you don't actually need that much to live on. On the other hand, be careful not to underestimate your expenses. Many high school students may think that $15,000 sounds like a small fortune when they're only earning $40 a week in a part-time job. But because they've always been supported by their parents, they don't realize how expensive it can be to live on their own. To avoid any shocks, estimate your living expenses *before* you choose a particular career. You'll need to consider housing, utilities, transportation, food, personal maintenance, entertainment.

When you total up your monthly combined expenses for the six categories, multiply that figure by twelve and you'll see the approximate amount of money your life-style requires. Note that this is on the low side, since it doesn't include taxes, savings, emergencies, major expenditures (i.e. furniture, stereo equipment), and little luxuries. This should give you an idea of how your yearly expenses for the kind of life you visualize would compare to the annual salary you could make in the health career that interests you. If there's a big discrepancy (namely, that your expenses far exceed your expected income), you have one of two choices: either to reject that career in lieu of a higher-paying one or to reevaluate your needs and see if you could trim your expenses. For example, you might consider managing without a car or sharing an apartment with a roommate.

Regardless of your reasons, don't feel defeated if you decide that a health career isn't for you. It's better to find out now, and spend your time and money training for a career that will make you happier. But if, after all your self-analysis, you're still convinced that you want a specific health career, you're ready to apply to schools that offer that curriculum. You've chosen your career and now you can pursue it. Congratulations on making one of the most important decisions of your life!

*Chapter 2*

# THE STUDENT YEARS

When you say that you're a college student, people immediately think you're having the time of your life. Beer blasts, partying till 2 in the morning, not a care in the world except for an occasional exam.

Nothing could be further from the truth. Granted, there *are* some students on campus who have nothing more on their minds than what they're going to wear to Friday night's dance. But for the students in my program, college is *hard work*. We're too busy studying and working to party all the time. When you have to be at a clinical placement at 7 in the morning, there's no way you can stay up late the night before. I'm not complaining; I've always wanted to be a nurse and I know I'm getting a great education here. But I'd be lying if I said it was easy. The pressure and stress can be incredible. I never knew how tough school could be until I started this program.

—Nursing student,
University of South Florida

Anyone who is currently enrolled in nursing or allied health studies or who has ever attended such a program will recognize the validity of that statement. There's just no getting around the fact that studying and training for a health career is a tough, demanding, and often exhausting process. At the same time, it is also stimulating, challenging, and ultimately rewarding.

## TRIALS AND TRIBULATIONS

Students in any major are quick to point out the demands and challenges posed by their course of study. Engineering students are convinced that their curriculum is the roughest. Medical students have no doubts that theirs is the most difficult program. Accounting majors are certain they have it harder than anyone else. Students of architecture, drama, dance, physical education, and philosophy firmly believe that their respective major is the most demanding.

Who actually does have it the hardest? The truth is that no college major is easy. Every academic program, from liberal arts to professional/technical majors, has its own unique characteristics which makes it more difficult in some respects and less demanding in others than another course of study to which it's being compared. The premed student might have to absorb more technical information than the elementary education major; on the other hand, the education major has both theoretical and practical skills to acquire. Chemistry majors have to spend long, rigorous hours in the lab, but dance majors spend equally long, exhausting hours at the barre.

There are, however, some aspects of nursing and allied health programs that make them truly more demanding and stressful than other college programs. For one thing, the vast majority of nursing and allied health students have had absolutely no previous exposure to the material. Unlike students majoring in biology, French, or English, nursing and allied health students are forced to deal with totally unfamiliar material. The biology, French, and English courses offered in high school give students a basic introductory background to these subject areas. Similarly, courses in psychology, history, or music provide a sound foundation for students who plan to major in one of these subjects in college.

But while it is true that some high schools have started to offer "Health Occupations" curriculums for students who anticipate a career in nursing or allied health, these courses are generic in nature, usually taught by a registered nurse. They do not necessarily give the student significant experience—either academic or practical—in respiratory therapy, medical records, or the other allied health fields. Consequently, students in nursing/allied health programs don't have any prior experience to fall back upon. Everything is new: the subject matter, vocabulary, professional skills and attitudes. The process of acquiring all this new knowledge and developing professional skills is an exciting one. It can also be formidable and even overwhelming at times.

Another difference between nursing/allied health programs and most other college majors is the emphasis placed on practical experience. The vast majority of majors do not require fieldwork experiences. As a rule, chemistry majors do not undergo an internship in off-campus laboratories. Practicums in major corporations, retail stores, and accounting firms are not generally a part of most business curriculums. Psychology majors usually aren't exposed to working with clients in any capacity during their undergraduate years. But, without exception, all nursing/allied health programs include a great deal of actual, hands-on experience working with people. This is a necessity, since a large part of the skills needed for health careers cannot be gained solely from a textbook.

But it is precisely this practical experience which places additional demands on nursing/allied health students. Whereas liberal arts students only have to contend with textbooks, memory work, term papers, and classroom lectures, health students have to combine all that with fieldwork which requires interpersonal skills and technical expertise. Dealing with people, especially those in physical or mental distress, presents unpredictable crises that you are expected to resolve. Performing procedures which require an integration of textbook knowledge, manual dexterity, and patient handling is infinitely more consuming than simply memorizing information from a book and reproducing it on a multiple-choice, true-false or essay exam. While absorbing new material, be it a foreign language or nineteenth-century American history, is never easy for most of us, having to assimilate it so integrally that it can be effectively applied to patients is an added dimension. You are *living* your curriculum, and your guinea pigs are people.

Yet another source of stress is the intensely *personal* nature of learning and performing a health care career. With most college majors, it is relatively easy to separate the learning *process* from the learner. Memorizing dates, reading textbooks, and taking written tests are all fairly impersonal and objective. When liberal arts students don't do well on a test, they usually don't take it too personally. They may tend to shrug it off with, "I didn't expect her to have so much on the role of the bourgeoisie."

But in nursing or allied health studies, it's harder to rationalize and view one's performance in a detached, objective manner, justifying a failure in terms of "The teacher did it." Because so much of health care courses involves *doing* and not just repeating facts, students in these programs tend to feel that their actual self-worth is bound up in their performance. If a procedure is performed incorrectly or difficulty is encountered with a patient, health care students are apt to berate themselves on a personal basis: "I'm clumsy," "I can't handle people well enough," "I don't have what it takes." Health students are quick to question and doubt their intellectual abilities, manual dexterity, personality, and everything else that goes into the performance of health care duties—actually, all of themselves—thus placing the blame for any "failures" on their innate abilities and personal characteristics, their entire selves, rather than on external factors, such as not enough time for studying or poorly designed tests.

Health care students can also find it somewhat of an identity crisis to have to adjust to their rather nebulous position of being somewhere between an uninitiated layperson and a full-fledged professional. From their first days, students are expected to internalize professional attitudes and behaviors; yet it is made clear that they are "only" students, with limited responsibilities and abilities. Regardless of how competent a student may feel, he or she is confined to a rigidly circumscribed role. The distinction between a nurse and a student nurse or a medical technologist and a medical technology student is not merely semantic. Students may be training for a health care career but they're not considered professionals until the day they graduate or pass their licensing exam. This kind of role ambiguity can be very disconcerting, and can put you in a bind. According to a first-year nursing student:

> Starting a new clinical placement is always difficult because you never quite know what's expected of you. There seems to be a very fine line between doing too little and doing too much. You can perform the same way in all your assignments, but one of your clinical supervisors might feel that you're overstepping your boundaries as a student if you take some initiative and try to tackle a difficult patient or new procedure on your own, whereas another supervisor might expect it of you and get upset if you ask for help right away.

A more subtle source of stress can be traced to the relatively low status of nursing and allied health studies on most college campuses, which we have mentioned. Engineering, business, and medicine are the elite majors, against which physical therapy, nursing, and medical technology don't rate. Fellow college students tend to be unimpressed by even a 4.0 average in nursing. Professors of the liberal arts and sciences often have negative stereotypes of health care students. They may feel that nursing and allied health students are only interested in the courses of their respective majors and therefore lack a true appreciation and aptitude for elective or required non-major courses. As one nursing student explains:

> I love art, but I felt really uncomfortable when I enrolled in a ceramics class. I worked just as hard as any of the art majors and actually became quite good at using the potter's wheel. But the instructor never seemed to take me seriously. When I would go to him for help with a problem, he would say things like, "Why are you so concerned about it? You're going to be a nurse, not a professional potter."

While many schools offer separate classes in introductory biology, chemistry, or physics courses for nursing and allied health students, others do not. Nursing students may find themselves taking an organic chemistry class with chemistry and premed majors. In such instances health students may feel that professors view them as inferior members of the class. According to one respiratory therapy student:

> Whenever I ask a question in my anatomy class, the professor becomes very condescending. He explains things to me as if I was a seven-year-old child. I have a pretty good background in science, but he treats me like I never even had a biology course in high school. When I tell people about the way he treats me, they think I'm being overly sensitive and even a little paranoid. They say that it's probably just the way he is. But they haven't seen the way he treats me and the other RT and nursing students in the class. He acts as though none of us are very bright, even though we all get excellent grades. The only students he seems to have any respect for are the bio majors and premed students.

An instructor in a graduate hospital administration program admits to an initial prejudice:

> For the past 5 years, I've taught a course in current medical issues and topics. The course is required for students in the graduate OT program as well as the MHA students. I was pretty apprehensive the first year because I didn't know quite what to expect. To be perfectly honest, I wasn't really familiar with the OT curriculum; I barely knew what OT was all about. Some of my colleagues kidded me about having a bunch of "basket weavers" in my class. I couldn't help feeling that I'd have to teach the class on two levels, addressing the topics on a superficial level for the OT students and on a more complex level to challenge the MHA students.
> After a month into the course, I saw that I couldn't have been more wrong. The OT students were actually more interested and capable than the students in my own pro-

gram. Whereas the hospital administration students just seemed to be marking time until they could go out and start earning the big bucks; the OT students seemed to genuinely care about all the health issues we discussed. I've gotten to the point now where I'd rather teach OT and other allied health students than those in the MHA program.

## MAKING THE MOST OF YOUR STUDENT YEARS

The student experience is always going to be a prerequisite for any nursing or allied health career. The nature of these fields necessitates intensive study and formalized training prior to assuming professional responsibilities. While it is possible to train for other occupations right on the job, health careers require 1 to 6 years of college and internship. With that amount of time as a student, it is important that these years be constructive and enjoyable.

Future health professionals need to keep the student experience in proper perspective. Training for a health career is serious business, and students have to tackle their studies with a high degree of determination and diligence. As we have noted, there is a vast amount of new material to be absorbed, as well as new skills and professional attitudes to be acquired, all within a relatively short period of time. The intellectual, emotional, and physical demands placed on health students can be enormous. Unfortunately, students often compound this stress by placing unrealistic expectations upon themselves and losing their perspective on the entire process of becoming and being health professionals.

While it is true that the most intensive learning takes place during the student years, learning doesn't end with graduation. If you feel that you need to learn all there is to know about your chosen field by the time you graduate, you impose undue pressure on yourself and set yourself up for inevitable disappointment when you fail to meet your goal. There simply is no way for you to acquire *all* the knowledge and skills you'll eventually gain with a few years of experience. The purpose of nursing and allied health programs is to prepare students to assume beginning professional responsibilities. No one expects a student fresh out of school to know as much or perform as well as a seasoned practitioner. Many employers formally differentiate between the new graduate and an experienced professional—ie., an occupational therapist "I" for a therapist with less than a year's experience, and an occupational therapist "II" for one with at least a year's experience. Naturally, there are different expectations, responsibilities, and compensation for the two levels. The more advanced level can only be gained through *experience*.

Even the best students are not going to know everything and perform flawlessly during the first few weeks on the job. It is imperative that students understand and accept this. Too often, health students burden themselves with unrealistic expectations. For your own well-being, you need to recognize the fact that, no matter how high your grades or how much time you spend studying, you're going to feel somewhat overwhelmed when you begin your first job. As one recent graduate in physical therapy notes:

> When I was in school, I studied much harder than anyone else in my class. I never allowed myself any time off; I was always at the library or at home cracking the books. While my classmates would get together socially, I was busy reviewing my notes and reading orthopedic and physical medicine journals. It wasn't just for the grades, although I did graduate at the top of my class: I honestly wanted to be a terrific physical therapist by the time I graduated. Looking back now, I see I went overboard with the studying and missed out on a lot of other experiences. Even with all that work, I still had a lot to learn when I started my first job. It wasn't until I'd been on the job for 6 months that I started to feel really comfortable and confident.

This is not to say that studying isn't important. It is, and it's your responsibility to learn as much as you can—but without sacrificing too many hours of sleep or doing without any social life. Keeping your student experience in proper perspective means that you'll study hard, that you'll learn all the required material and even go a little beyond, but that you won't make yourself miserable if you encounter difficulty in some areas or when you feel like you're never going to learn it all. You *will* learn it, but it will take time. Don't burn yourself out by trying to absorb it all right away.

Also, maintain a rational perspective on grades. You should do everything you can to earn good grades, but keep in mind that they're only a reflection of your performance as a student. Getting all A's as a student does not necessarily mean that you're going to be an outstanding practitioner when you graduate. Every nursing and allied health instructor or clinician can tell you about someone who received the best grades in academic courses but did poorly in clinical work. Instructors frequently believe that many "straight-A" students have certain personality characteristics that prevent them from functioning effectively with other people. In many cases, students who receive fair-to-good grades but have a well-rounded, integrated personality, life-style, and outlook can perform their professional responsibilities better than the class grind who studies to the exclusion of everything else. As a radiologic technology instructor sizes it up:

> There are always one or two students in every class who really excel in the academic portion of the program. While some of these students have an enviable ability to quickly grasp the physics and technology, others have to plug away to get their good grades. You have to give these students credit for their diligence and determination, but I often find myself wishing that I could make them understand that grades aren't all that important. They'd probably be shocked if they knew that some of their instructors just got mediocre grades when they were in school, but it's true. Grades, especially those for academically oriented courses, just don't tell the whole story.
>
> A lot of students with extremely high grade point averages don't do all that well in the clinical setting. Some have difficulty applying their book knowledge in practical situations. Others aren't able to handle patients very well. They may know the right answers on a multiple-choice test but never seem to know how to relate to other people. After all that solitary studying and striving to get the best grades,

these students frequently have trouble getting along with their peers. They don't know how to work effectively with someone else; they've never had experience with being a team player.

Remember, also, that once you get out, no one knows or cares what your grade point average was. The C student and the A student are equals in the work setting. The A student doesn't get more responsibilities or a larger salary than the B or C student. All that concerns your supervisors and patients is that you've successfully completed your studies and can competently perform those duties for which you are hired.

Try not to be in awe of your instructors. Give them the respect they've earned, but see them as people. They don't know everything—just more than you do! Don't be afraid of them; they're being paid to help you learn. Don't endow them with magical powers. They're not omnipotent and they can't bestow knowledge and skill. Learning a health profession is not a passive process; the student needs to be actively involved. All that the instructor can do is work in conjunction with you, the student, to help you master the essentials. It usually helps to remember that your instructors were once students, too. They were just as confused and overwhelmed as you are now. They received the same training that you're currently getting. Seeing them in this light will help you relate to them more successfully—as human resources, not gods.

During your student years, try to get as much practical experience as possible. While all health programs incorporate practicums, these are often placed towards the latter part of the program. By then students are deeply entrenched in the program and may not be inclined to withdraw or change majors, even if they find that the clinical aspect is not for them. If your program does not include any clinical exposure at the outset, seek it on your own through volunteer or paid work. Ideally, this work will be related to your chosen field, i.e., transporting patients to respiratory therapy if you plan to be a respiratory therapist or working in the dietetics department if you want to be a nutritionist. While it's true that this experience won't give you a complete picture of what it would be like to actually be a respiratory therapist or dietician, since you'd have only limited duties and responsibilities, it will still provide you with firsthand knowledge about the general work that these health professionals are involved in. Those high school students we mentioned earlier, who decided they wanted a health career because they "like working with *people*" or "want to *help others*," once they get into the clinical portion of their studies, may find that it's more than they bargained for and that they really don't like working with *sick* people, and their "help" doesn't work any dramatic change.

Education is never a waste. Even if you decide not to continue with a specific health program or opt not to actually practice the profession, the time spent in your studies would still be worthwhile since you have gained new knowledge and learned a lot about yourself in the process. But because education can be expensive, it's in your best interests to make sure the career for which you're training is what you really want. Relevant work experience (either paid or voluntary) will help you in this regard, as well as adding another dimension to your resume. Having additional practical experience can give you an edge on your classmates when you're all looking for that first job. So even if you feel overwhelmed by all your courses in the first few months, try to do a couple of hours of volunteer work each week. In addition to giving you contacts and references when you're ready to start looking for a job, it also will convince you that a health career is right for you—or, just as importantly, let you know if it's not. An hour or two away from the books can be bracing to your mental health and contribute to the perspective we've been talking about.

Do whatever you can to enhance the image of your chosen occupation. All too often, other students are barely aware that there are nursing and allied health programs on campus. Contact between health students and liberal arts majors can be extremely limited, particularly during the junior and senior years when almost all the courses are exclusively within the major curriculum. Whenever possible, try to take a course outside your major. Even if it's only on an audit basis, it will bring you into contact with students from other majors who you probably wouldn't get to meet under normal circumstances. Since one of the purposes of college is to broaden your horizons, relating with a variety of people is a learning experience that helps you to grow as a person. Being with students from other majors can help to relieve stress and burnout by allowing nursing or allied health students to be exposed to different viewpoints and concerns rather than limiting their focus to only what is relevant to their own curriculum. As a dental hygiene student recalls:

> The best thing I ever did last semester was to enroll in a filmmaking class. I know it seemed kind of strange to my classmates in the dental hygiene program, since movies and teeth have nothing in common, but I found myself feeling too confined and somewhat bored when all I took were dental hygiene classes. There wasn't a whole lot of room for any creativity and all my classmates ever talked about were scaling, root planing, and fluoride treatments. I really needed some sort of outlet. I didn't want my whole life to be dental hygiene. While I'm never going to be a Hollywood director, the class was a lot of fun. I met lots of interesting people and really felt stimulated and challenged. It may have taken away a few hours of studying time each week, but it was well worth it. The film class gave me a much needed break from the daily grind, recharging me for my "real" studies.

Try to avoid the vicious circle that health students often find themselves caught in when taking a class outside their major. As we have noted, many students in other majors feel that people who choose to major in a health science aren't as bright, dynamic, or ambitious as those who major in business, law, medicine, or one of the natural sciences. Health students sense this and are often reluctant to fully take an active role in non-major classes, preferring to maintain a low profile. But this only serves to perpetuate the stereotype, further convincing students in other majors that health students are inferior academically, intellectually, and socially. For your own sake, as well as the image of the nursing and allied health professions in general, don't fall into this trap. Everyone, regardless of their major, academic background, or previous experiences, has something worthwhile to contribute to a class, and health students are no exception. Just as you plan to become an active, contributing member of society, so you should be an active, contributing member of your class, even if it's in a course as unrelated to your major as ancient Egyptian history or Elizabethan poetry. These classes might have no direct bearing on your major course work or your future job duties, but it's important to you, to your classmates and to the instructor that you make the most of them.

Similarly, participate in as many campus activities as you possibly can. It's fine to belong to a club or society sponsored by your major, but don't restrict yourself to just that. When you graduate, you'll probably belong to other clubs and organizations besides your professional association, so why not enlarge your horizons while still a student? While students should take part in extracurricular activities related to their intended professions, there's no reason why they shouldn't also be involved in activities that enrich the campus as a whole or that allow them to express their other interests. Students majoring in speech pathology can be active in student government; students in nursing or nutrition can work on the campus newspaper in a variety of positions; medical technology students are free to join any political, religious, social, or avocational group that interests them.

It's best not to enter school with rigid plans for your future. Many students are convinced that they know exactly what they want to do after graduation even before they take their first class. After volunteering on a pediatric unit while in high school, a first-year nursing student may feel certain that she wants to work only with children. A physical therapy major may be sure that he wants to specialize in geriatrics after seeing a therapist rehabilitate his grandmother after a stroke. But quite often, these early decisions aren't the best ones because there hasn't been enough exposure to all the possibilities. Although she enjoyed playing with the children on the pediatric ward as a volunteer, the nursing student may find it difficult to actually perform nursing procedures on her small patients. She might eventually find that she prefers dealing with adult patients who are better able to understand and tolerate pain and discomfort. The physical therapy major may discover that he finds sports medicine much more challenging than geriatrics. It's important to keep an open mind about all the different specialty areas of your intended profession and try to get experience in as many as possible. As an occupational therapist recalls:

> When I started school, I was a hundred percent sure that I wanted to specialize in psychiatric O.T. Since my father is a psychiatrist, I've grown up with an interest in mental illness. It seemed natural for me to go into psych. O.T. I never even considered going into any other area of O.T. I concentrated on learning all I could about psych. while not paying a whole lot of attention to the physical disabilities and pediatric portions of the curriculum.
>
> But when I graduated, there weren't any job openings in psych. I had to take a job in a children's hospital and I've been there ever since. It's okay now, but the first few months were incredibly rough since I didn't have that great a background in pediatrics. I wish now that I had been a little more receptive to other areas of O.T. while I was in school.

Resist the temptation to prematurely map out your entire career before you've adequately explored every option. Remember that there's absolutely no need to lock yourself into anything while you're in school (or even during your first year or two after graduation).

Make the most of your student years. While the amount of time you'll spend as a student seems insignificant compared to the number of years you'll actually practice your profession, your years as a student are extremely important since they lay the foundation for the rest of your career. Work hard, learn a lot, and enjoy doing it.

*Chapter 3*

# THE FIRST YEAR(S)

I couldn't wait to begin my first job. During the last couple of months of school, all I could think about was graduating and starting to work. I had really enjoyed school but I was counting the days until I'd be out on my own being a "real" therapist. As far as I was concerned, it was going to be wonderful not to have to worry about grades or an instructor looking over my shoulder.

But I soon discovered that it wasn't quite as wonderful as I thought it would be. I felt too unsure of myself to enjoy being on my own; I found myself wishing that I still had a supportive instructor to turn to. My supervisor was okay, but it wasn't the same sort of relationship I had had with my professors. There was very little feedback unless I did something terribly wrong. I almost wished I was still getting graded so I'd know how I was doing.

—Respiratory therapist,
San Diego

All students look forward to their first job. Regardless of their major, they are anxious to finish school and start applying what they've learned. They seek professional challenges as well as a regular paycheck.

But the transformation from a student to a working professional is not always smooth. Students aren't guaranteed a job the moment they graduate; they must actively search for one that both utilizes their qualifications and fulfills their expectations. Once they find it, they discover that the working world is quite different from the college campus. Unless they learn to adjust their behavior and thinking to the new situation, recent graduates may experience shock, anxiety, or even depression.

## GETTING YOUR FIRST JOB

### The Job Search

Nursing and allied health graduates have it easier in some respects than liberal arts majors. Unlike students who have majored in sociology or English, health majors know exactly what they want to do after graduation. They made the decision 1 to 6 years earlier.

Some of the more trying aspects of hunting for a job in the business world don't affect the health graduate. Whereas liberal arts majors typically face the catch-22 of not being able to get a job because they don't have experience and not being able to gain experience because they can't get a job, employers in the health care field are willing to hire new graduates. Since hospitals and other health care employers are assured of a certain degree of entry-level competence, thanks to the graduate's training and licensure/certification/registration, they are comfortable with hiring people without any experience. The brand new nurse, technologist, or therapist may lack some of the skills of the seasoned professional, but the employer knows that the new professional has mastered the basics and demonstrated the personal attributes necessary for successfully performing the job.

But while health graduates don't have to worry as much as liberal arts majors about types of jobs to consider, career strategies, and an inaccessible workplace which demands experience, they are narrowed down to a more limited sphere of potential employers. The employment options of nursing and allied health graduates are restricted to nursing positions in hospitals, clinics, home health agencies, or doctor's offices. Therefore, health graduates haven't the same kind of flexibility as other college graduates in planning their job searches.

This is not to imply that the job outlook for nursing and allied health graduates is discouraging. If there is a smaller number of health care positions available than business openings, there is a proportionally smaller number of job seekers for these positions. On almost every college campus today there are many more students majoring in business than in medical technology or nursing. Consequently, there usually isn't the intense competition among health graduates for jobs as there is between liberal arts majors. With a little persistence, most health majors manage to find a job shortly after graduation.

Your first step in hunting for a job should be to decide where you'd like to live. Some new graduates are determined to find a job in their hometowns. For some, this is a wise decision since they know what to expect from the area and probably have established a good many contacts over the years. Being able to live at home can save money, an important consideration if your first salary is on the low side, and can ease the often stressful transition from student to employee. On the minus side, job opportunities can be very limited unless you live in a major metropolitan area.

Other new graduates set their sights on employment in their college town. As with the hometown setting, you have a built-in advantage of having established contacts and the area. But openings can be competitive because a large percentage of graduates also decide that they'd like to remain in their college town. If you're convinced that you want to continue living in the area, at least be flexible about the exact location. There may be more opportunities in a town an hour's commuting distance away. This would still allow you to frequently enjoy all that the college town has to offer, while increasing your odds of finding a job.

If you have no compelling practical or personal commitments to tie you down to a specific area, you have virtually unlimited possibilities. But make sure that you consider the actual *job* in question and aren't just focusing on the locale. As an occupational therapist notes:

> I chose my first job for all the wrong reasons. I had always dreamed of living in southern California, so I was determined to find a job there when I graduated from school. I took the first job that came up, both to be sure that I'd be able to move to Los Angeles and also to avoid having to go to a bunch of other interviews. I barely paid attention to the facility when I went for my interview; all I could think about was catching some sun later and looking for an apartment. But after I had been there for a few weeks, I began to realize that I'd made a big mistake. The administrator had some unrealistic expectations about how many patients I could treat each day; they wanted me to run an assembly line where the patients were wheeled in and out every 5 minutes so they could bill as many patients as possible for therapy. I should have thought twice about working in a nursing home in general and this one in particular.

When considering jobs in distant locations, ask yourself the following questions:

*Is it the job or the location that attracts me?*
If this particular job was located in a city which wasn't nearly as appealing, would I still be interested in the position?
*Have I done my homework about the cost of living in that area?*
Do I know what kind of housing is available and what the rentals run, whether I'll have to pay for my own heat (which can be as high as rent), whether there's local bus service if I don't have a car? Have I tried grocery-shopping in the local supermarket, and compared prices? Without this "hands-on" knowledge, salary figures can be misleading. Salaries in Alaska, for instance, sound unbelievable, but the cost of living is at least equally high. Salaries in small southern towns may seem unacceptably meager, but the cost of living can be so low that your discretionary income (the amount you have left over after paying fixed, necessary expenses) can be substantial.
*Have I toured the area till I have a pretty good idea of what it would be like to live there?*

This does not mean just checking out the beach. Look at the available housing that you can afford, checkout transportation facilities, what the weather is like year-round. If you love reading and skiing, make sure that there's a decent library and ski slope. A small rural town may be picturesque, but if you're a sophisticated type, you may have a hard time making friends with your views and interests, finding your favorite magazines, or any entertainment in the evenings. A large metropolitan city might have unlimited cultural life but you may always be yearning to get out of town for sports and outdoor recreation.

*Are there other job opportunities nearby if this job doesn't work out?*
If you decide after 3 months that you can't stand your new job, it would be extremely costly and disruptive to move again. If you're in a very small town with only one hospital, your chances to switch jobs while remaining in the same locale might be very limited. Before you get yourself into a spot like this, either make very sure that you're going to want to stay a while in your new job or that you'll have enough of a financial reserve to move if need be.

After tentatively deciding on a few places where you might like to live, try to determine what sort of work setting would be most personally satisfying for you. Hospitals, of course, are the foremost employer of health care workers, but even among hospitals there's substantial variation. Large hospitals, particularly those that are part of a national chain, usually offer excellent fringe benefits such as comprehensive health coverage, tuition-aid plans, day care, stock benefits, or profit-sharing plans. Smaller hospitals, nursing homes, doctors' offices, laboratories, clinics, agencies, and private practices may not offer benefits as extensive. Some may not offer a pension plan, for example, but this may not be a consideration since the majority of new graduates don't stay in their first job long enough to get vested in their employer's pension plan. Larger hospitals may have more opportunities for advancement, but smaller facilities and organizations that have the potential to grow can also provide opportunities to move up.

There are other considerations besides money and advancement. Larger hospitals may be better staffed and equipped. If you're in a highly technological field (such as radiation technology, medical technology, respiratory therapy, or physical therapy) which places a heavy emphasis upon electronics and machinery, you may find it to your advantage to work in a setting with state-of-the-art equipment. This avoids demoralizing shock that new graduates experience when they go from the modern equipment they were trained on to obsolescent equipment. Roles are more narrowly defined in a large health care setting; this may or may not be an advantage over smaller settings. Knowing exactly what your duties are and being able to follow them to the letter is less anxiety-provoking than having to be more fluid and self-structured in your duties and responsibilities. Larger facilities will better enable you to specialize in a specific area, whereas smaller facilities help you to be more of a generalist. You have to decide which is right for you in the long run. As a physical therapist describes it:

> When we graduated, my best friend accepted a job at a 600-bed teaching hospital while I took a job at a 150-bed community hospital. They had her deal almost exclusively with hand patients, while I treated a little bit of everything. I have to admit that I envied her. It sounded so prestigious to be specializing in something like hand therapy rather than being a jack of all trades. After about 18 months, we both decided we were ready to for a change and started to look for other jobs. Due to my varied experience, I found a new job much more easily than she did. General hospitals weren't that interested in her because her experience and expertise was limited to just hand patients.

You may also wish to reflect on whether you'd be happier in a proprietary or a nonprofit situation. Idealistic recent graduates may be uncomfortable in profit-making facilities since it may seem that there is more of an emphasis on the bottom line than on quality patient care. On the other hand, employees may feel frustrated by the ever-present lack of funds in nonprofit facilities and feel that it compromises patient care.

Once you've pinpointed what sort of job you'd like and where you'd like to live, your job search begins in earnest. The most obvious starting point is the classified ads. Your local newspaper is fine if you want to stay in the general vicinity, but you'll need to go to a large newsstand or public library to look at an out-of-town paper if you're setting your sights on a distant city. Keep in mind that almost every other job seeker is also searching through these ads; competition will vary depending on the position but can be intense.

Avoid taking the ads at face value. The "best" ads do not necessarily correlate with the most desirable jobs. Just because an ad is long, detailed, or cleverly written does not mean that the job it's trying to fill is any better than a position advertised with briefer, more run-of-the-mill copy. The job ad only reflects the writing skills of the person who wrote it. Hospital A may have a personnel director who writes more appealing ads than the personnel manager at Hospital B, but that doesn't automatically mean the jobs at Hospital A are any better than the jobs at Hospital B. In fact, cynics might suggest that conditions and pay at Hospital A might not be all that great and that's why in desperation they've hired someone who has a flair for words.

Learn to read between the lines of want ads. "Experience preferred" means just that. Experience may be preferred, but it's not *required*. Apply for these kinds of jobs even if you may not be the employer's prototype of the ideal candidate. He or she might not get any other applicants who come any closer to fulfilling the criteria. Don't be misled by salary quotes. "Salary *to* $27,000" does not guarantee you $27,000 if you get the job. Since you don't have any experience, you should expect to start at a few thousand less than the top salary.

Answer a classified ad immediately, both to create an efficient impression, and because the job may be filled fast. Follow the ad's instructions exactly. If it says "Mail resume; do not phone," then you have to rely on the mail. Don't let anyone persuade you that real go-getters show their eagerness by then phoning to make sure their resume got there. Health care employment doesn't want that kind of go-getter.

The usefulness of newspapers in generating job leads goes beyond the classified section. Just reading the local news can turn up some ideas. If you see that a hospital has just announced plans for expansion or that a new nursing home will be opening, you have an opportunity to get in on the ground floor and avoid all the competition that you'd have to fight if the job were advertised. Write a letter immediately that expresses your interest in this vitally needed new facility and enclose your resume.

The phone book can also be helpful. Using the telephone enables you to contact many employers in one day. Granted, you won't get a lot of positive responses; unless you're in a field noted for chronic shortages of personnel, many of the employers you call won't have any openings. But you may find a potential employer who knows of a job opening that will be occurring within the foreseeable future. If your timing is right, you may contact an employer who has a letter of resignation sitting on his or her desk and just hasn't gotten around to calling in an ad to the newspaper. S/he may be very happy to schedule an interview with you to avoid the time and expense of composing and placing an ad.

When you're told over the phone that there aren't any openings, you're not likely to take it as a personal rejection since the employer is a faceless stranger who can't see you. In answering an ad that gives a phone number you may be nervous when making your call. To avoid getting flustered, you may want to have a written script in front of you. Don't read from the script verbatim, but use it as a prompt to remind you of what you want to say. Write down a brief summary of your qualifications, and jot down questions you'd like to ask. This way you won't forget an important point.

If you're told the job has been filled, you can ask if you could send a resume to be kept on file in case of future openings. Some facilities will invite you to come in and fill out an application "just in case something turns up in the future." There's certainly no harm in having a resume or application on file, but don't expect anything much to come of this. All too often, applications are filed away and forgotten. By the time an opening materializes, applications may have been discarded. This is especially true when you send your resume to the personnel department. Whenever possible, try to file your resume with the person who's in charge of the department where you'd be working. If you're an occupational therapist, for example, send your resume to the Director of O.T. This person would be more likely to actually read and remember your resume.

General employment agencies may not have many health

care positions to place their clients into, but there are agencies that specialize exclusively in the health field. If you live in a large metropolitan area, you may find some of these agencies listed in the Yellow Pages. In addition, these agencies may advertise in your professional journals and newsletters.

These employment agencies can be extremely helpful if you're moving to a distant city. However, you'll need to keep a few things in mind when dealing with an agency. Most reputable agencies are "fee-paid," meaning that the employer foots the bill when the agency successfully places a candidate in the position. Since employers pay the bill, the agency is working for them and not you. They're not necessarily going to look out for your best interests. Their goal is to place as many people as possible. Some "counselors" may be quite aggressive in encouraging you to take one of the jobs they're trying to fill. Make sure you're not pressured into anything; make up your own mind about the jobs they're pushing. Also make sure that you don't get railroaded into purchases like resume or interview "workshops" or vocational tests. You don't need a vocational test; you've already pinpointed what it is you want to do. As far as learning how to write a resume or interview successfully, the agency should coach you on this without any charge to ensure that you'll make the best impression and be placeable.

Almost every college or university has a placement office whose function (usually free) is to assist graduates in getting jobs. Unlike private employment agencies, college placement counselors don't have a direct financial stake in getting you a job, so some of them might not be overly concerned to place you. Nonetheless, they may have substantial listings of job openings, particularly if your alma mater is known for having a strong program in your major. Employers from all over the country may have written to the placement office or your major's department office, seeking graduates to fill their vacancies.

## The Resume

Resumes are important even for first-time job seekers with no experience. Quite often they provide the first impression your prospective employer will form about you. Remember that a resume must "sell," and not merely describe you. Make sure it looks very polished. Have it professionally typed. Typesetting is another (but very expensive) alternative. Photocopies should be clean and sharp, on white 8½ x 11″ paper. If you read a general career guide, you'll often see offbeat resumes on colored paper mentioned with other attention-getting measures, but this is appropriate only for creative fields like advertising. In the health field, you'll need to follow traditional decorum or you'll appear unprofessional. Health care employers aren't looking for mavericks; they want employees who can abide by their rules and policies.

The following guidelines provide some do's and don'ts for composing a resume.

*Personal information.*    Begin the resume with your full name, address, and phone number. Note your registration and licensure numbers, if applicable. This should be the extent of your personal information. There's no need to give your age, sex, race, height, weight, or marital status. Do not attach your photograph; your appearance has nothing to do with your qualifications for the job.

*Career objective.*    Provide a brief statement that describes your professional aspirations. This can be as general as "To begin a career as a registered nurse." It could also be more specific, i.e., "To utilize my psychiatric nursing skills in a community mental health center." Naturally, your career objective should correlate with the job you're seeking. If you're a physical therapist who's interested in working in home health care *or* sports medicine, don't note this on the same resume. To avoid sounding indecisive, write two separate resumes, one with the goal of working in home health, and the other addressing your interest in sports medicine. This way, you can aim a specific resume to a corresponding position.

*Education.*    As a recent college graduate with no pertinent job history, you'll want to start with your educational background. List the names and locations of the colleges from which you earned degrees. Include the year you received your degree. State your major and any academic honors or awards you received. While your prospective employer will have a good idea of the kind of courses you took within your major, you may want to list elective and non-major courses that may have some relevance. If, for example, you're a nursing graduate who took a special topics course in gerontology and you're applying for a job in a nursing home, it would be appropriate to list the course since it emphasizes your interest in geriatric nursing. If you're an occupational therapist who happened to take a lot of craft courses as electives, you may want to include a statement such as "Additional elective courses in ceramics, weaving, and jewelry making" if you're applying for a job in a psychiatric facility.

*Work experience.*    While you obviously don't have any full-time, paid, professional work experience, you can list your field-work experiences, clinical affiliations, and internships. List the names, addresses, dates, and highlights of your experiences— i.e., "performed 50 serum cholesterol levels," "worked with laryngectomy patients," "ran an exercise group for Parkinson's patients." State your responsibilities in a brief but comprehensive manner. Above all, state them honestly. Don't inflate your duties and responsibilities; your prospective employer will probably see right through it, knowing that you couldn't possibly have done all that as a student, and you'll lose all credibility. Worse yet, in the rare situation that exaggeration is taken at face value, you could land in a job that's frighteningly over your head.

*Other information.*    Additional information that doesn't fit into any of the previous categories can be included here. You may want to list professional associations you belong to, or special skills not previously mentioned, such as fluency in a foreign language or computer skills. Some job hunters include personal interests like hobbies, sports, or travel, but usually this sort of information is not pertinent in any way to the job you're seeking.

*References.*    Don't give the names, addresses, or phone numbers of your references; just put "References available on request" at the foot of your resume. When you know you're really interested in a job and that the prospective employer is truly interested in you, give references from whom you've gotten permission. Permission assures your getting strong references from former professors and clinical instructors, and gives you an opportunity to refresh their memories about you and your accomplishments.

*Cover letter.*   The cover letter may be even more important than the resume, since the prospective employer will read it first. Whereas your resume can be a Xeroxed copy, you'll need to submit a typed, individualized letter for each position you apply for. Use the standard business format, including your name and address, as well as the name of the person to whom you're writing. Usually you can get a name over the phone by inquiring, "for the purpose of addressing a letter." Use the salutation "Dear Sir or Madam" when you cannot get a name.

Compose a brief (one page or less) letter to suit the position in question. Introduce yourself by mentioning what position you're applying for, how you heard about it, and why you're interested in it. Briefly explain what your qualifications are. Since you don't have any significant work experience, your qualifications are simply that you've successfully completed your training and are now registered, certified, licensed, or eligible for registration/certification/licensure.

End the letter by saying that you're enclosing your resume. Do not say, "If you have any questions, please do not hesitate to contact me". This is trite, and sounds snotty. The employer will take it for granted that since you're interested in the position you'd be willing to answer any questions. Instead, end the letter on a positive note: "I hope to hear from you."

Some career counselors recommend saying something like, "If I do not hear from you by the middle of next week, I will call you to discuss setting up an appointment." Career counselors tend to be strong on "assertiveness" because so many clients who seek career counseling are very uncertain personalities. But, if the basic "*We'll call you*" rule is disregarded, what employer would have time to run an office? And, you don't give him a deadline by which he should reply. (It's not *unheard* of to get a response a year later—and the timing may be right!)

Definitely, in the health field, employers try to fill vacancies as quickly as possible. It's certainly permissible to express warm interest in the job, but stick to conventional routes (the U.S. mail). If you're applying for an advertised position, the employers will contact you if they're interested and when they're ready to schedule an interview.

## The Interview

*Application.*   You'll usually be asked to fill out a job application before your interview. To make sure it presents you in the best possible light:

> Read the application once from beginning to end *before* writing *anything.*
>
> Print neatly.
>
> Give a telephone number where you can definitely be reached during the day. (Make sure your four-year-old nephew won't be answering the phone.)
>
> Include your pre-married name on the application if you're a recently married woman using your husband's last name.
>
> Fill out all items. Use N/A for "not applicable" if a question doesn't apply to you (i.e., military service). Do not write "See resume" in any blanks. Even though your educational or job history *is* on your resume, fill it out anyway. The purpose of the application is to conform to company screening procedures.
>
> Put "Negotiable" in the blank under salary expectations, or the minimum you can work for.

*Your Appearance.*   There are many books that can teach you how to dress for success. All these books are geared to the business world, however, and aren't always appropriate for the health care field. In fields where uniforms are worn, it may not be necessary to wear a suit, regardless of whether you're male or female. A sport jacket or even just a crisp shirt and tie may be acceptable for men, and a simple wash dress can be fine for women. You don't need a briefcase as a prop, although you will want to bring an extra copy of your resume. Traditional standards of good taste should prevail in grooming: conservative clothing, natural makeup, no perfume, minimal jewelry, conventional hairstyle.

*Body Language.* Make sure your handshake is firm and confident. Smile appropriately. If you never smile, you'll seem nervous and unpersonable; if you smile constantly, it may appear that you're not taking anything seriously. Utilize frequent eye contact, but shift your gaze from time to time to avoid making your interviewer uncomfortable by staring. Refrain from smoking, and don't have a pack visible in shirt pocket or handbag. Of course, don't chew gum.

*The Interview Itself.* It's normal to be a little nervous when interviewed, but try to remember that an interview is really nothing more than a conversation which will enable you both to give and seek information. Look upon it as an opportunity to convince your employer face to face that you're the best person for the job.

Nursing and allied health graduates have an advantage over business majors when it comes to interviews. In the business world, interviewers may deliberately create a stressful atmosphere just to test how the applicant can handle pressure. Applicants for business positions may be forced to "sell" themselves in a more competitive, less supportive atmosphere than that in which health care applicants are interviewed. Unlike the more subjective business world where applicants have to prove their qualifications, nursing and allied health graduates are considered to be qualified applicants by virtue of their training and registration/licensure.

If you're interviewed by someone from the personnel department, don't expect anything more than a cursory screening. The personnel interviewer doesn't know anything about your field and isn't capable of asking any sort of probing questions about your skills and qualifications. At the most, he or she will skim your application/resume, checking your educational background, and registration/licensure/certification. You may be asked for the names and addresses of references, and will probably be told about the general working conditions and employee benefits. At this point, you'll usually be turned over to the head of the department under which your position falls. This person (who most likely would be your boss should you get the job) will handle the in-depth interview.

A good interview will be a give-and-take situation. Many inexperienced job seekers expect that the interviewer will be in total control by asking the questions while they assume a passive role of merely answering the questions. Try to remember that it's in your best interests to be an active, equal participant in the interview process. Your first goal of an interview is to present yourself as an alert, motivated, energetic person who would be a good candidate for the position. At the same time, you also need to make sure that you could be reasonably happy in the position. Neither goal can be fully accomplished if you just sit back and let the interview happen to you.

On the other hand, you don't want to take over the interview. It's one thing to be confidently assertive, but quite another to be brashly aggressive. Let your interviewer set the tone and then follow his lead. If it is clear that he is well organized and is following a set agenda, don't switch the flow of dialogue; add information that is closely related to the question you've been asked. By all means, sell yourself by adding points that weren't covered and ask questions that remain unanswered, but do this after the interviewer appears to have concluded the structured interview.

But not every interviewer is organized, efficient, and in control. Some will be just as nervous and ill at ease as you, obviously unsure of how to take charge of the interview. In these cases, the ball's in your court and it's up to you to score a few points for yourself. If the interviewer is so reticent that you encounter an awkward silence, it's permissible to use a conversational icebreaker. It can be appropriate to make a complimentary observation about the facility, as long as it's sincere. If your first impressions about some aspect of the facility are favorable, it may be worth noting. Looking up something about its history may give you a fitting conversational gambit. After all, the interviewer is an employee of the facility and he or she probably takes pride in working there. It's easier for him or her to feel drawn to you if you seem enthusiastic about the possibility of working at the facility.

Most interviewers have a few standard questions they ask any interviewee. The following list, though not all-inclusive, mentions some of the most frequently asked questions. Read both the questions and the suggestions for answers, then formulate an answer that would work well for you.

*Can you tell me something about yourself?*

Describe your education and training, stressing what is most pertinent to the position. Mention vital influences that drew you to your specialty.

*Did you enjoy school?*

"*Especially—*"Since, of course, you didn't love everything and everybody, think in advance of positive things to mention—a marvelous professor, a particularly exciting course, lab, or field-word—unusual opportunities your school offered. Come across as if regarding yourself as lucky. Mention *advantages* you enjoyed, not deprivations. Don't refer to controversies in which you were involved, or tangling with the Dean. Say school was a great experience and you learned a lot, but now you're eager to start working so you can begin to use it.

*What is your greatest strength?*

Don't worry about sounding immodest. Make the most of this opportunity to convince the interviewer that you'd be a good choice for the position. Appropriate answers might be: your ability to learn quickly; your commitment and willingness to work hard; your high energy level; your ability to handle stressful situations; your flexibility in relating to a wide variety of patients.

*What is your major weakness?*

It's possible to turn this question around, answering in a way that portrays you in a positive light. Find a "good" bad quality, such as your tendency to take things too seriously or your impatience with people who don't do their share of the work that needs to be done.

*Why do you want to work here?*

Don't say "Well, I need a job, and I heard about this," "It's handy for me to get to," or, "My friend works here." Touch upon something specific to the position or facility—i.e. "Your hospital

has an excellent reputation for providing quality patient care"
or "I've heard that you have a lot of opportunities for continuing
education."
*What are your short-term and long-range goals?*
or,
*What do you expect to be doing in 2, 5, or 10 years?*
Many new graduates try to impress their interviewers with their
ambitions and aspirations, answering these questions with statements like "I would hope to be promoted into an administrative
position after a year or so of working here." But statements like
this can backfire. The interviewer may write you off as being
likely to quit the job after a short period of time if a promotion
didn't come through. If the interviewer had to wait 10 years for
his own promotion to an administrative or supervisory position,
your confidence may seem naive and immature. Make sure your
goals are realistic. It may be best to say that your immediate goal
is to learn as much as you possibly can and that you'll crystallize
your long-term goals once you've had more experience. Mention
only those aspirations that directly relate to your professional
field. If you dream of becoming a singer or taking a couple of
years off to travel around the world, keep these goals to yourself.

There are some questions which, because of their highly
personal and irrelevant nature, are illegal for an interviewer to
ask. These include:

> your religious affiliation.
> your marital status or plans.
> whether you have children or plan to.
> what your spouse/parents do for a living.
> whether you own or rent your home or apartment.
> your political views or organizations to which you belong.
> your financial status.
> whether you're in debt.

If an interviewer asks an illegal question, you don't have to
answer, but make sure you refrain in a tactful manner. You can
also skirt the issue by indirectly answering the question—i.e., "My

biggest priority right now is my career" when asked if you plan to marry or have children in the near future.

Sometimes, through no fault of your own, an interview may not go well. If the interviewer has to deal with frequent interruptions like phone calls, it may be hard for either one of you to get back on track. Interviewers are human too and may be preoccupied with their own personal problems to the point where they can't properly conduct the interview. If you feel that you haven't had a fair chance to present yourself favorably (due to your interviewer's attitude or your own extenuating circumstances, such as not feeling well), you may want to call the interviewer back the next day and see if you could reschedule another interview. If your dissatisfaction about how the interview went stems from something the interviewer did or did not do, you'll need to be especially tactful. Be careful not to blame the interviewer. Simply say something like, "After thinking about our interview, I realized that I didn't cover my qualifications as fully as I intended. Would it be possible for me to come in for a short second interview?" If you weren't feeling well, note this, with something like, "Because I wasn't feeling at my best yesterday, I may not have appeared as interested in the job as I am. I'd like to let you know now that I was really impressed with your facility and I'd definitely like to be considered for the position."

If you're not offered the job on the spot, follow up the interview with a thank-you note to the interviewer. Thank him for the time spent touring the facility and answering your questions. Make it clear that you liked what you saw and would like to work there. After you do that, there's really nothing else you can do— except to sit by the phone and wait for the call that lets you know you've got the job!

## MAKING THE MOST OF YOUR FIRST YEAR(S)

The first year or two after graduation is as important to a professional career as the first few years of childhood are to later physical, intellectual, and emotional development. The first years provide the foundation for everything that transpires thereafter. This is the time that the neophyte develops into his professional self. The transformation doesn't just happen overnight; it occurs gradually over the course of time. Some health care workers may feel comfortably settled into their professional selves within a few months, while others are just beginning to reach that stage after 2 years. Regardless of the actual time it takes, all health professionals are faced with the process of becoming acclimated to their new roles and responsibilities.

Students who have just graduated from college often find it difficult to adjust to the working world. After spending only a few hours a day in classes, with breaks in between, it can be hard to get used to having to work steadily at least 8 hours a day. Having to arrive at work at 9 o'clock every morning is quite different from being able to roll out of bed 15 minutes before an 11 o'clock class. A 15-minute coffee break once or twice a day can't compare with hanging out in the student union for much of the day.

Health students may have less of an adjustment to make than students in other majors when graduation comes. Rather than picking an easy, convenient schedule, most students in health majors have to follow a rigid schedule that involves long hours in clinical assignments, classrooms, and libraries. Since all health students have had clinical training, they've already experienced the working world. They have less of a culture shock than psychology or history majors when they begin their careers. But even so, there are adjustments to make. Being a health care professional *is* different than being a health care student.

It is quite common for any new professional to feel overwhelmed at first. New health care professionals are especially subject to this feeling. Suddenly they're on their own, away from the protective cocoon of their training program, and they're responsible for the health of other human beings. Whether their job is preparing specimens for laboratory procedures or instructing patients on how to take care of a colostomy, everything that health care workers do is going to have impact in some way on their patients' well-being. Sometimes this impact is indirect, as is the case with medical records or medical library personnel, but ultimately it all affects the overall delivery of health care.

When the new graduate realizes the enormity of his responsibilities, panic can strike. New professionals in the health care field may feel that they haven't been adequately prepared by their schools to assume these responsibilities. It's easy to blame professors or colleges for the feeling of inadequacy, but new graduates need to realize that no one is really to blame. Your program did the best it could to prepare you to assume an entry-level position in your chosen field. The only alternative would be to expand the length of the program, but most students would be reluctant to invest additional time and money beyond the 1 to 6 years they've already put in after high school. Besides, even if the training period was doubled in length, it still wouldn't solve the problem. Students could train from here to eternity, but they're still going to feel somewhat unprepared and unsure of themselves when it comes time to really be on their own. There's always going to be that transition from student to full-fledged professional, and no amount of education is going to alleviate the "growing pains" that new professionals will feel.

It may help to realize that everyone experiences that feeling of insecurity. New graduates in every allied health and nursing field all feel inadequate at first. You may look with awe at the more confident, experienced professionals and wonder if you'll ever reach that point, but what you're not seeing is how these self-assured, seasoned professionals *got* that way. They didn't start out with that level of expertise; that's something which can only be acquired through experience. Believe it or not, they once felt very much like you do right now.

You may be able to find an experienced professional in your field who's willing to show you the ropes. Many people enjoy sharing their knowledge and welcome the opportunity to teach and "mold" a novice. In the corporate world, having a mentor who acts as a career coach can be an important factor in achieving career success. Mentors aren't quite as crucial in the health care field, but they can still be valuable. A mentor can steer you, offer encouragement, tip you off to problem areas, give you inside information, and introduce you to people who might prove to be important later on in your career. Finding a mentor isn't always easy. You can't just pick someone whose style you admire and make a nuisance of yourself. This kind of relationship can only develop when the timing and personalities are right. There has to be reciprocity. But if you find a coworker or supervisor with whom you're compatible and whom you respect, you can get across that you feel you have a lot to learn from this person and really appreciate any help that she or he is willing to give. Be quick to acknowledge a suggestion: "Oh, thanks so much for telling me!" "I'm really glad to know that."

Remember that you can't learn everything overnight. Even the most voracious reading isn't going to instantly result in the kind of knowledge that can come only from years of experience. As a registered nurse notes:

> I felt like I didn't know anything when I first started working. I felt like an imposter, like I was just masquerading as an R.N. Those 4 years of school just didn't seem like they had prepared me for everything I needed to do and know.
>
> After being really uptight the first few days on the job, I decided I needed to do something about it. I spent all of my breaks and even a couple of hours after my shift was over in the medical library, trying to read all the medical and nursing journals. When I got home from work, I spent hours reading and rereading all my old textbooks.
>
> But after about 6 weeks of this routine, I found myself burning out. I just couldn't keep up that pace any longer; I'd start work each day feeling both physically and mentally exhausted. All that studying and reading wasn't doing a thing to improve my job performance or level of confidence. Gradually, I learned to relax and let things develop on their own. It took quite a few months, but eventually I began to feel comfortable. I discovered that even without all that extra work, I had learned quite a lot just by being on the job.

No one could fault you for wanting to learn more about your profession. One of the qualities of a true professional is commitment to keeping up with current trends and practices. What you learned in school is only the beginning. There's no way that you can be an effective health care worker throughout your entire career without refreshing and expanding your knowledge base. Reading professional journals, books, and attending continuing education opportunities are all crucial. The trick is to strike the balance between how much learning is stimulating and clarifying and how much is overload. Make sure you do at least a little studying on your own. There is no set length of time that's right for everyone; it depends on your field, educational background, level of expertise, and motivation. Setting aside a couple of hours for study each week seems to be a realistic goal for most people. This should give you enough time to at least keep up with your professional journals.

But don't make the mistake of the nurse who devoted almost every waking hour to learning all she could about nursing. This only leads to burnout and is in no way beneficial for your physical or emotional health. Your free time should be spent in ways that will refresh you, and help you grow as a person and not just as a health professional. There's no reason to feel guilty about going bike riding after work or curling up with the latest novel. In the long run, you'll bring more verve to your job if you spend the majority of your nonworking hours in activities that are a complete change from your career.

Every new employee worries about making mistakes. No health care professional is immune from making a few blunders during the first months, and it's a safe bet to assume that you will, too. It's all right to make mistakes on your first job, provided they're not major ones that endanger a patient's life or health, cost a lot of money to repair, or result in a legal jam. There's no excuse for careless or stupid mistakes, but honest mistakes which stem from a lack of experience will usually be tolerated your first months. Above all, don't make the same mistake twice. The fact that a mistake was tolerated the first time does not mean it's acceptable for it to occur again. If you honestly learned from the mistake, you'll be careful not to repeat it.

Work on developing an aura of self-confidence. This may be hard to pull off at first since you're bound to feel unsure of yourself much of the time. But it's important to appear in control of the situation, especially for your patients' sakes. They may know that you're inexperienced but will accept you as a professional if you give the impression that you're secure in your abilities. If you act confident, you'll be perceived as competent by your patients and coworkers alike. This doesn't imply that you should exude the sort of brash cockiness that turns people off; what you need to cultivate is a quiet self-assurance that you have what it takes to handle the job. You may not know everything, but you've been trained and certified as having the level of competence that's expected of someone with your experience. The fact that you've passed your training courses and your registration exams reflects well upon you. Your professors and the members of a licensing body felt that you have the personal attributes and expertise to handle your job. Although you may not be able to do things as well as some of your more advanced coworkers, you can take pride in your accomplishments even at this early point. As an occupational therapist relates:

> All the other OTRs at my first job were excellent therapists. I was particularly impressed with their splint-making abilities. Whenever a splint needed to be fabricated for a patient's hand, they just whipped out the material, started measuring, and 20 minutes later they had completed a splint that looked good and fit properly. But the first couple splints that I tried to make were a disaster. I was all thumbs with the material, getting my fingerprints all over it, and it didn't even fit the patient! After over an hour of struggling with it and wasting a lot of material, I finally had to ask for help from one of the therapists. She did it so effortlessly that I felt really bad about not being able to do it myself. I was really discouraged about my abilities (or lack of them, to put it more accurately), but the therapist who had helped me with the splint told me that I was being too hard on myself. She said that my first attempt at splinting was actually a lot better than the first splint she had made as a new therapist; in fact, she said that I showed a lot of promise!

**Learn to be assertive.** There are numerous books available which can help you to become more assertive. Don't confuse assertive behavior with aggressive behavior. Assertiveness is merely a way of communicating in an honest, open, direct manner that takes into consideration both your own personal rights *and* the rights of others. Whereas acting aggressively usually means you're trying to win at someone else's expense, assertive behavior attempts to satisfy *your* needs while making sure you don't hurt anyone else in the process.

Assertive behavior does not come naturally to many people. Since the vast majority of health care workers are female and society has historically taught women to be passive, it is not surprising that nursing and allied health professionals frequently find it difficult to be assertive. Their schooling and professional socialization have traditionally geared them to speak in a low, doubtful voice, agree automatically, and accept whatever prevails. Health care workers have been expected to completely disregard their own needs while attending to the physical and emotional needs of others. They weren't supposed to be concerned about rewards such as money, prestige, recognition, and satisfactory working conditions. But things are changing. While health professionals are still dedicated to the needs of their patients, they've learned that there's nothing wrong with making sure they get their due.

As a beginning health professional, you're not in a position to seek significant financial remuneration for your work. Your lack of experience will place you at the lowest end of the salary scale and there's very little that you as an individual can do about increasing your salary and benefits. But you do need to learn to be assertive about ensuring that you work under the best possible conditions. It's unfortunately quite common for beginners to be given work assignments that are the most arduous and amount to an overload.

Many workers who are just starting out feel that they're being taken advantage of by their bosses or by the system in general. The most common complaint is the tendency for new workers to be assigned the "worst" jobs. Laboratory workers may be delegated the most tedious procedures to perform; nurses may be assigned patients who are high-handed, who insist on smoking in bed, or who resist prescribed treatment; speech pathologists may be given the most severely aphasic stroke patients. If you find this happening to you on a consistent basis, you'll need to counter it in an assertive manner. Too many inexperienced, young health professionals are reluctant to speak up and are afraid to make waves. They get indoctrinated into the philosophy that they need to "pay their dues" by doing the heaviest jobs that are foisted on them by their older, more experienced peers.

But this way of thinking is unwarranted and detrimental to

your professional well-being. You've already paid your dues simply by going through your professional schooling and passing the exam that qualified you for your first job. Your lack of seniority should not automatically condemn you to all the scut work or to the most trying patients. Let your supervisor know that you would appreciate a more varied workload. In a firm but tactful manner, inform him or her that you would like assignments similar to those of your coworkers. If your supervisor feels that you're not ready to handle some of the tasks you're interested in, work together to develop a plan to help you gain these skills within a predictable timespan.

In some instances, new health professionals may find that, while they're not necessarily assigned to the roughest duties, they seem to be confined to serving the juice, wheeling patients to the lounge, or filling the water jugs. If you feel that you're capable of more complicated and specialized jobs, be assertive about requesting more challenging assignments. Remind your supervisor that you won't be able to grow professionally unless you're allowed to experience a variety of duties and responsibilities. You may need some help with the more difficult tasks at first, but you'll soon gain proficiency and confidence in your abilities. Don't make the mistake of carving out a comfortable niche for yourself during the first few months and then never wanting to jeopardize that security by taking on new challenges. While it's possible (and even probable) that you might run into some hitches and won't score instant success, you'll at least be on your way to developing some new skills and will augment your image as someone who can handle more complex procedures. When you're just starting out, no one is going to pass judgment on you if you have trouble with something you've never done before.

Don't be afraid of your supervisor. This kind of stagefright stems from a misperception. Try not to be in awe of his or her power, prestige, or position. If you can learn to look upon the role of a supervisor in a positive light, you won't be as likely to be intimidated by this important person. Rather than seeing him or her as the person who is waiting to see what you're going to do wrong, realize that your supervisor's real role is ensuring that you perform as efficiently and productively as possible. You are both in this together. The two of you are working towards the same goal: achieving your potential as a health professional. Your supervisor isn't an adversary who is out to pounce on you, but a resource person who can help you.

The need to be assertive isn't restricted to just your dealings with your supervisor. Assertiveness is also necessary in your interactions with colleagues and patients. The scope of this book does not permit a detailed discussion of how to develop assertiveness, but there are several books available on the subject:

Angel, Gerry, & Petronko, Diane Knox: *Developing the New Assertive Nurse*. New York: Springer, 1983.

Bloom, Lynn, Coburn, Karen, & Pearlman, Joan: *The New Assertive Woman*. New York: Dell, 1975.

Gerrard, Brian A., Boniface, Wendy J., & Love, Barbara H.: *Interpersonal Skills for Health Professionals*. Reston, Virginia: Reston, 1980.

Greenleaf, Nancy P.: *The Politics of Self-Esteem*. Wakefield, Massachusetts, Nursing Digest/Contemporary Publications, 1978.

Herman, Sonya J.: *Becoming Assertive—A Guide for Nurses*. New York: Van Nostrand, 1978.

Stevens, Kathleen R. (Ed.): *Power and Influence*. New York: Wiley, 1983.

All health professionals need to be able to get along with their coworkers. It's particularly important for new graduates to interact effectively with the people they work with. Without the help and support of their coworkers, new health professionals will find their first years very difficult. A team mentality is definitely required of workers in the health care field, but this may not come naturally to you as a new graduate since college required you to work on your own for the most part. The learner has to be pretty much of a loner. Academic programs usually foster more competition than cooperation among students; they do very little in the way of teaching you how to be a team player.

Functioning as a member of the team is a skill which you'll need to acquire in the early days of your career. No book can give you explicit instructions on how to do this, since the personalities and circumstances you have to deal with are unique to your situation and may be completely different from those of another reader. But it may be helpful to consider the experiences of other people so that you can avoid the mistakes they made during *their* first years. According to one registered nurse:

> Things didn't go too smoothly at the beginning of my first job. Looking back now, I realize that I was to blame for most of the difficulties I had with the people I worked with. I was so anxious to prove myself that I came on too strong. I really wasn't very sure of myself, but I didn't want to show it, so I acted overly confident to the point of being cocky and brash.
>
> As the newest and youngest R.N. on the floor, I was determined not to let anyone take advantage of my age, inexperience, and lack of seniority. In my second week into the job, one of the other nurses asked me to switch shifts with her since she had some out-of-town relatives she wanted to take out to dinner that night. Not wanting to set a precedent or to get a reputation for being a pushover, I refused. This resulted in all the other nurses ostracizing me as much as they could and really backfired on me when I got an invitation to a party I was dying to go to and no one would switch shifts with me.
>
> I made a lot of other mistakes, too. I was extremely critical of the way our hospital and our unit were run. I never missed an opportunity to point out what was wrong with the way things were done and then I couldn't understand why people felt offended by my criticisms. It took me a while to realize that a lot of the nurses had worked there for years and had very strong emotional ties with the hospital. They identified very closely with the unit and the hospital, so they took a lot of my criticism personally, even when I didn't mean it as a reflection upon them.
>
> I also let everyone know time and time again that I was a college graduate and was more up-to-date than anyone else on the latest procedures and techniques. Needless to say, this didn't win me any friends among the other nurses

who had gone through a diploma program years ago. But it didn't take long for me to find that I needed their help. I soon discovered that there was quite a lot I didn't know and quite a few situations I had trouble handling. By that time, though, my coworkers weren't anxious to bail me out of any problems I ran into. When I finally was forced to swallow my pride and ask for help, they'd say things like, "Didn't they teach you that in college?" or "Gee, don't ask me, I'm just an old-fashioned nurse without a degree. I thought you were the expert."

One of the toughest aspects of adjusting to the work world is the lack of feedback. Recent graduates in all fields feel a blank in going from frequent comments from professors to the sporadic remarks offered by their supervisors. The fact is that it doesn't occur to most bosses to let you know when you're doing well; they only point out your mistakes and weaknesses. In many cases, a paycheck is the only positive feedback that a worker gets. If you absolutely find it impossible to function without getting any reaction, talk to your supervisor to see if your work can be evaluated on a more regular basis. Perhaps your supervisor can schedule 10 minutes for you every few weeks to discuss your performance. It may be possible to make up a rating sheet that will let you know how you're doing in several different areas such as the various technical procedures or the handling of patients. Be aware, though, that some supervisors will take the attitude, "This is no school. You've been to school. Nobody lets me know how *I'm* doing unless something goes wrong." You will need to learn how to critique your own performance and to provide your own reinforcement for a job well done. It's often the only thanks you'll get, and it can be the best.

New professionals in almost every career field experience another kind of "reality shock" when they make the transition from school to work. They often find there's a clash between what they've been taught and the way the real world operates. The realities of the workplace may not match and can even violate the principles and practices learned in school. They quickly see that the textbook responses to idealized situations are difficult, if not impossible, to utilize under the constraints of the system.

New health care professionals are particularly vulnerable to the stress that occurs when they perceive the discrepancy between the values learned in school and the realities of the workplace. Not only do the new graduates have the physical stressors of learning to adjust to shift work and 40-plus hour weeks, but they also are forced to deal with the obstacles that prevent them from providing the type of patient care they expected to deliver. New health care workers often feel bitter toward their schools when they realize that they weren't adequately prepared for the realities of the work environment and may also become angry at the system for so often operating in an inefficient or inhumane manner.

Job-hopping isn't the answer to resolving the conflicts and frustrations of your initial years of a health career. The "perfect" hospital or employment situation doesn't exist. No matter how many jobs you try, you're not going to find a position or work environment that provides you with total satisfaction and no hassles. Nonetheless, the time will come when it's a good idea for you to move on to another job. There's no set length of time to stay in your first job. Some people will benefit by changing jobs after 6 months, while others will do better by remaining in their first job for a couple of years. You'll know it's the right time for you to move on when:

> another job offers you more *opportunities* for you to expand your expertise and further develop your skills.
>
> you can make *significantly* more money or receive far better benefits in another job. (Be careful about leaving just for a few extra dollars. It may not be worth it to leave a job you enjoy if a slight increase in pay isn't really going to change the quality of your life. Remember that there are no guarantees that you'll like your new job once you get into it.)
>
> a new job will actually be a *promotion* for you by allowing you to supervise others or work more independently, providing you're ready for this.
>
> a new job will offer you the chance to gain *skills in a different area* of your field, thus adding to your total knowledge base and ability to function within a wide range of settings.

you're terribly bored with your job. (Make sure it's just the job you're bored with, and not your profession in general.)

working conditions at your present job are intolerable and you're positive that other jobs offer *better conditions*.

you're unable to resolve major and continuing conflicts with your supervisor even though you've tried hard to improve your relationship with him or her.

Your second job should offer you opportunities to build on your skills and acquire new ones. In many cases, this will be a lateral move without a salary increase or higher status. Some workers may even find it wise to accept a slight cut in pay if a new job offers more promise for the future than your current one. Lateral moves are much easier to make during the early years of your career before you become too specialized and somewhat restricted to a certain niche in your field; but do use discretion in switching jobs. While it's not expected that a worker will remain in the same job for 30 years, you don't want to hop from job to job so frequently that your resume will imply that you have no stability.

Your first years may not be easy, but there's no short cut or way around them. Years later, you'll either look back on them as a necessary evil or as a positive experience in which you learned a great deal. If you'd prefer being able to see them as the latter, you need to do everything within your power to make the most of these early years.

# Chapter 4

# THE MIDDLE YEARS

When I was being interviewed for nursing school, the Admissions Committee asked me what I hoped to be doing in 5 to 10 years. I really didn't know what to do years later; my only concern at that point was to get into the nursing program. But thinking that I'd better sound like I was ambitious, I said that I would like to be in an administrative position by then. I was accepted into the program, so obviously that must have been what they wanted to hear.

After graduation, I couldn't wait to start nursing. It was every bit as fulfilling as I thought it would be. Even after 3 years, I still loved working with patients. Yet, in the back of my mind, I kept remembering my interview. It had sounded impressive to say that I planned to go into administration. It would be less than ambitious not to want to rise up the nursing hierarchy. I couldn't help thinking that only an undynamic and unmotivated person wouldn't be interested in moving up and moving on to bigger and better things.

So I grabbed whatever promotional opportunities came my way. When an opening came up in Utilization Review,

I eagerly applied for it. But once I was in that position for a few months, I realized I had made a mistake. I hated it! I missed the direct patient contact and the camaraderie with my coworkers. I was determined not to quit, though, because the Utilization Review position was a highly visible one that put you on the fast track for other promotions. My career strategy paid off. After 4 years in the UR position, I made it to my management. Now I'm a full-fledged administrator . . . and hating every minute of it. I don't like dealing with budgets or personnel policies. Being a staff nurse was much more satisfying to me. I'd love to go back into direct care, but I'm not sure I want to give up my present salary and status. I would have thought that I'd have all the answers after 7 years, but at this point, I don't really know *what* I want for the rest of my career.

—Registered nurse,
Alexandria, Virginia

Career confusion and uncertainty are not restricted to the first years of work. Workers in the middle years of their careers can experience a lack of direction about where they're headed. Although they have acquired a few years of experience, they still may have unresolved questions about their careers. In addition to the universal concerns shared by workers in all stages of their careers, there are some issues that are unique to the middle years. It is then that workers typically commit themselves to a specialty area of the profession. The middle years are also those with the greatest potential for career growth. Workers who have "proven" themselves during their beginning years now begin to look forward to promotions and advancement opportunities. At the same time, the excitement and novelty of the first years begins to diminish. Work becomes more routine and not quite as challenging as it was initially.

It should be noted that there are no definite boundaries of the middle career years. Since your career is a continuum of experiences, there is no formal cut-off point that separates the first years from the middle years. Some workers may have become fully acclimated to their jobs and mastered virtually every skill within a couple of years. Others take longer to adjust and to acquire advanced skills. Even after 4 or more years of experience, they may still feel like beginners. In general, however, your middle career years will begin after about your third year and will continue until you have approximately 10 years to go till retirement. During these years, you'll realize the peak of your abilities as a health professional. You'll have grown into your job and your role as a health care provider. In addition to increased confidence in your abilities, you'll have developed an expertise that can come only with experience. It's also likely that you'll need to resolve one or more of the following dilemmas.

## SPECIALIZATION VERSUS GENERALIZATION

Most health care workers tend to specialize in a specific area of their fields by the time they complete their third year of work. Some decide what specialty area they want during their training programs; a few choose their specialties before they begin their education. But many workers need several years' exposure to the various aspects of their fields before they can decide what area appeals to them the most. If this appears to be the case with you, make sure you don't prematurely lock yourself into a specialty area. All too often, health care personnel get into a specialty by default. As a registered nurse reports:

> I wasn't sure what area of nursing I wanted to go into when I graduated from school. I knew a little about all the different areas, but not enough to be positive that any one area was the right one for me. I chose my first job on the basis of its location and salary rather than on the type of nursing it was. It happened to be in pediatrics and I stayed in the job for 4 years. There was a lot I liked about that particular job, so I was pretty satisfied with pediatric nursing. When I got married and moved away, it seemed logical to seek another pediatric nursing job. After 3 years at that job, I wasn't all that happy with it and wanted a change. Since I had friends who did industrial nursing and really enjoyed it, I thought I'd like to look into employment with a big corporation.

But I soon found that it wasn't going to be easy to switch from peds to occupational nursing. Some employers seemed to doubt my sincerity in wanting to change specialty areas. They questioned my motives and wondered whether I'd really be able to "switch gears" from working with children in a hospital to working with adults in a factory setting. It seemed that I was going to be forced to remain in pediatrics for the rest of my career. When I finally landed the sort of position I was looking for, I quickly discovered that I much preferred working with adults. I hate to think how close I came to being in pediatrics for the rest of my career just because my first job happened to be in that area.

Even if you're positive that you've chosen a specialization that's absolutely right for you, it can still be helpful to try a different aspect of your health care field. Working for a year in another area of your profession can be looked upon as a professional working "break." If you find yourself becoming stagnant, different surroundings, duties, and patient populations can help revitalize you. There are new things to learn and new procedures to master, thus presenting a professional challenge that may no longer be present in your current situation.

Consider the possibility that it may be better for you not to commit yourself to one specialty for your entire career. Most health care fields appear to be leaning towards splintering off into various specializations, but there will always be room for generalists as well. There often seems to be more prestige and increased salary potential for those who specialize; but there are other rewards for those in general practice. Work can be more stimulating because of the diversity of the patient population and the greater variety of professional responsibilities. The likelihood of burnout may be decreased for generalists, since they aren't confined to a narrowly circumscribed work world. In addition, generalizing reduces the chances of "growing *out*" of your career. As you change and mature during the years, there is the possibility that the specialty area you once enjoyed no longer seems to suit you. As a physical therapist relates:

I've been specializing in sports medicine for the past 9 years. At first it was really exciting. I felt like a pioneer in a relatively new field and there was so much to learn. But now it's become very mundane and predictable. I see the same few injuries over and over again. When I first started, I was really into sports. It was easy for me to relate to people with athletic injuries. But, 9 years later, I'm a different person. I'm not so interested in sports anymore. The athletes have begun to bore me; they strike me now as being too self-absorbed and obsessed with sports. Many of the injuries could have been prevented with a little bit of common sense. My practice is not as gratifying as it used to be. It's not that sports medicine has changed; I'm the one that's changed. As I got older, I acquired different interests and values. I probably won't get out of the specialty since I own my practice, but I can't help thinking that I should have gone into general hospital practice like the majority of my classmates. Most of them still seem pretty happy. They get to see all different types of patients and perform a variety of procedures, whereas I'm pretty much stuck doing the same few things over and over again with the same type of clients.

This is not to say that specializing is wrong for everyone. Developing expertise in a certain aspect of your field can definitely have its rewards. Specializing usually carries more prestige than being a jack of all trades. If status is important to you, you may be happier in a prestigious specialty area. Just as physician-specialists have higher incomes than those in general practice, so do specialists in the nursing or allied health fields. There may also be more job opportunities in specialties with critical shortages of personnel.

All other concerns aside, there is really only one basic consideration you need to keep in mind when deciding whether to specialize or generalize. Only you can know whether you'd be happier knowing a lot about a little or a little about a lot. It's up to you to know yourself well enough to answer that question as honestly and realistically as possible.

## MOVING UP VERSUS STAYING ON

Once you are beyond the beginner category it's time to think about what direction you want the rest of your career to take. Are you hoping to advance your career by moving up into a supervisory or managerial position, or would you be happier staying on and doing the same sort of work you're currently involved in? It's a decision you're going to have to make for yourself; no one can do it for you. You can procrastinate indefinitely about this decision and take the attitude of "whatever happens, will happen," but only if you're not interested in being in control of your career. Full control is never possible, true. We're all bound to some degree by external circumstances and events. But coasting passively along can engender a sense of dissatisfaction that is embittering and disabling in itself.

Advancement into a position with more responsibility seems like a logical career progression for workers with good job performance and several years of experience. After mastering the demands of their own jobs, they may be ready to tackle new challenges. But there are two problems that confront these workers.

The first problem is the lack of opportunities for many qualified workers. Consider this example of a hypothetical therapy department with 23 therapists. There are two full-time speech therapists and one part-timer, seven full-time occupational therapists, and 10 full-time physical therapists and three part-timers. The two occupational therapists and four physical therapists with less than 2 years' experience are not qualified for supervisory positions. The four part-timers aren't eligible for any promotions. That leaves 13 experienced therapists who conceivably would like to advance in their careers. Unfortunately, there are only three positions above the staff therapist level. There's an occupational therapist supervisor and a physical therapist supervisor, plus a rehabilitation services department head. But three positions between 13 potential candidates means that 10 therapists won't have any opportunity to advance beyond the staff therapist level. Some of those therapists might quit their current positions to work at a different facility, but they still might find that the odds continue to be stacked against them. Because there will always be more staff positions than supervisory/administrative positions, not everyone who aspires to move up will have anywhere to go.

The second problem is that supervisory/administrative positions require unique skills that may be far different from those needed for most nonmanagerial health care jobs. Many health care workers feel that they have what it takes to be a manager because they've done well as a health care provider. But this doesn't necessarily follow. Supervisory and administrative positions utilize skills and talents that aren't typically taught in many health curriculums. Moreover, performing the duties of a health care provider doesn't develop those skills needed for a managerial position. It can be a sharp change from health care provider to manager. The needed skills can usually be acquired after awhile, but the personal characteristics and temperament of some health care workers may be at odds with what is needed for effective management. Calmness and fairness are essential. Greater formality may be desirable. You may need to curb your spontaneity. Verbal expression must be clear and definite, without sounding officious.

Most health care workers choose their respective fields because they feel that the work will be meaningful and enjoyable. What appeals to them is the opportunity to work with people in need and perform specific highly skilled tasks. They don't envision themselves sitting behind a desk behind piles of paperwork or disciplining workers with poor job performance. Had they had a special interest in management, they would have opted for a degree in business management rather than one in radiology technology, respiratory therapy, social work, or nursing. But, they were interested in an entirely different set of responsibilities. Yet the only way to experience any sort of career advancement is to give up those duties that drew them to the health care field in the first place. If they want more pay and prestige, there's usually no choice but to abandon direct patient care and move into management.

Some health care workers find that they really don't miss the patient contact when they get promoted. They feel that their new duties are challenging and rewarding on their own terms. Other health care workers who have moved into management aren't happy in their new roles. They dislike the bureaucratic machinery that an administrator is part of and would prefer hands-on patient care. As a registered nurse reveals:

> I was thrilled when I got to be the Director of Nursing. At thirty-four, I was the youngest D.O.N. the hospital had ever had and I couldn't believe my good fortune. But I quickly found that I wasn't cut out for it. I hated the petty politics and the length of time it took to get any problems resolved. I never felt like I could really make my own decisions. I could make suggestions, but ultimately, the hospital administrator and the board of directors had the final say. I was especially uncomfortable with being forced to place more emphasis on the bottom line than on the quality of patient care. It seems everything boiled down to money, but that's not a philosophy I'm comfortable with.
>
> I was doing some paperwork one day when it suddenly occurred to me that I really wasn't a nurse any more. I had become nothing more than a paper-pusher and a figurehead. What I was doing wasn't much different than what I'd be doing as an executive in a large corporation, except that I was making a lot less money doing it in the hospital than I would be in the business community. But that wasn't where my heart was. After a lot of soul-searching, I decided to resign. I took a job with a home health agency where I'm working as a real nurse again and I have no doubts that I did the right thing.

Don't automatically assume that you should move into management simply because it seems like the next step after a few years of experience. Make sure you truly do have leadership ability and that you'd be happy in exercising it. While management styles can be as varied as the people who serve in these positions, there are several personal characteristics that are essential for effective leadership. If you can answer the following questions affirmatively, you probably have a good chance of succeeding in and enjoying a management position.

> Do my coworkers and supervisors usually respect my *judgment?*

Do other people look to me for *direction?*

Am I generally *confident* about my skills and abilities?

Am I able to make sound *decisions?*

Can I see into the future and visualize the long-term *results* of my decision making?

Can I set aside matters of *personality*, and make *objective* decisions?

Can I be as *flexible* as the situation requires?

Is it more important for me to be *respected* than to be *liked* by my colleagues?

Do *I respect* my coworkers' abilities? Do I understand that I'd need to *delegate responsibility* to them if they were my subordinates and that I couldn't do everything myself?

Would I be able to handle *a change in my relationships* with my coworkers? Would I not let it bother me that my coworkers would probably stop considering me a personal friend and buddy and view me instead as a boss?

Can I provide *my own reinforcement* for a job well done?

Is *my own opinion* of my work more important to me than anyone else's?

Am I considering a career move into management because I genuinely feel I'd enjoy the duties and responsibilities, and not just because I want to *escape* from the daily stresses of direct patient care?

Am I fairly familiar with what my duties and responsibilities would be if I became a manager?

Am I positive that I don't want to be in management *just* because of the prestige and salary?

If you come to the conclusion that you definitely are interested in moving into management, there are several things you must do. You have to make yourself visible. Make sure you're noticed. *Speak up* at meetings and *volunteer* for special projects such as conducting inservices and workshops. Become *active* in your professional association. *Conduct yourself as a professional* at all times, including presenting a professional appearance. Finally, and perhaps most importantly, let it be known that *you're interested in advancing.* Don't just assume that the-powers-that-be will know that you'd like to move into management. Be candid about your interest in moving up and don't hesitate to apply for appropriate openings as they arise.

## STAGNATION VERSUS GROWTH

One of the biggest problems facing health care workers in their middle years is how to keep growing professionally. After a few years on the job, workers have acquired all the skills and knowledge necessary to the basic practice of their profession. They then have the choice of remaining at that level for the rest of their careers or taking action to further their professional expertise. As has been noted, it can be comfortable and definitely easier to maintain yourself at level. But it's infinitely more stimulating and satisfying to expand your skills and knowledge, and to feel that you're in the swim of a fast-moving world.

The most obvious way to grow professionally is through continuing education. Most health care fields offer a wide variety of advanced courses which are sponsored by health care facilities, colleges and universities, and professional associations. There are also courses and seminars offered by proprietary companies. You'll need to critically evaluate the contents, objectives, and credentials of the faculty before you sign up for any course. Some will be worth your while, whereas others will prove an exasperating waste of your time and money. Whenever possible, audit a single session, or at least talk to people who have taken the course. When you do find a course that seems promising, do everything you can to prepare to get the most out of it. Review the subject matter before the workshop or seminar and come prepared with a list of questions about anything you have problems with. Be an active participant, and not just a passive observer. Think about what's being said and really digest it. Ask questions, enter into discussions. Also try to make some new professional contacts while you're there. Network, rather than just hang around with the same colleagues you see every day at work.

You can also take college courses that aren't specifically related to your career field. You don't have to be a psychologist to benefit from various psychology courses; any worker who deals with people needs to understand human behavior. Similarly, sociology courses can also be helpful. Most health professionals will also find that philosophy and religion courses can help them to develop their own personal philosophies about their work and about life in general. Management courses can be appropriate for workers who are currently in supervisory or administrative positions as well as for those who aspire to them. Communication, writing, and public-speaking courses can enable health care workers to express themselves more effectively.

Another very meaningful avenue for professional growth is research. Every health care profession encourages its members to engage in research to increase their current bodies of knowledge. You'll be advancing both yourself and your profession if you participate in research studies. Many health care workers find the idea of research intimidating, but it doesn't have to be ponderous. You might not have the scholarly tools to do a research project from hypothesis to summation, but you can work on a single step, such as collecting data. If you lack confidence or experience in doing research, contact your professional association, former instructors, or colleagues with more of a bent in this direction.

Whenever possible, tackle new aspects of your job. Look for new procedures or different ways of doing things. In addition to making your job more interesting, mastering new challenges will also add to your self-esteem.

Working with students can help to renew your professional enthusiasm. Health care students are eager to learn and often ask thought-provoking questions that will stir you to review your texts and to acquire new knowledge. Just as you were once a student who needed to do clinical internships, young students are coming up now in need of the same opportunities you were once offered. Being in charge of a student will give you supervisory experience and will also expose you to new knowledge in your field.

Some health care workers frequently change jobs in an attempt to avoid professional stagnation. Rather than remain in the same job, with the same people, doing the same things, they look for a change of pace by switching work environments. When the new environment becomes familiar and routine, they change jobs once again. Each job change does offer new experiences and opportunities for professional growth, but only on a temporary basis. After a certain point in your career, you need to carefully evaluate the advantages and disadvantages of changing jobs.

One of the most important considerations in your middle years is becoming vested in a pension plan. Some employers don't offer any pensions at all. Even if you work for them for 30 years, you could retire with nothing but a plaque commemorating your years of faithful service. Employers who do provide pension plans generally require that employers work for at least 5 years before they can become vested in the plan. Keep this in mind when considering a job change every couple of years. If you switch that often, you will have escaped the monotony associated with remaining in the same job for years on end, but your retirement income may suffer as a result.

Although the middle years can be associated with some difficult career decisions and concerns, they can still be a joyful experience. You can continue to grow professionally and to assume new leadership roles. Most of all, you can feel good about yourself because you've shown that *you have what it takes*. You're no longer a beginner; you've acquired all the skills and knowledge needed to successfully perform in your profession. Whether it's 5 years or 15 behind you now, this is a triumph of which you have every right to feel proud.

*Chapter 5*

# THE LATER YEARS

When I was just starting out as a physical therapist, I was fortunate enough to work with several older therapists who had almost 60 years of experience between them. I was able to learn a great deal from them and still appreciate everything they taught me. I really felt that I lucked out in my first job. If I had had to work with less experienced therapists, I don't think I would have learned half as much those first couple of years.

I'm no longer a novice. After 40 years, I guess I qualify as an older, experienced therapist. But the younger therapists don't have a whole lot of use for me. PT is so different now than it was when I went to school that the other therapists regard me as a fossil. It doesn't help, either, that I'm not as strong as I used to be. I have to get assistance with most transfers and gait training, and some of the younger therapists resent having to help me.

I used to love PT, but times have changed. I'd retire tomorrow if I could, but I can't until my youngest son finishes college. So all I can do is make the best of it and count the days until retirement.

—Physical therapist,
Portland, Maine

The last 10 years or so of your career should be more than just marking time until you retire. Your last years of work should allow you to continue to grow professionally. This is a time in which you can use the considerable experience and wisdom you've gained over the years to make a significant contribution to your health care field.

There are concerns that may arise in your final years of work, such as those noted in the poignant testimony of the Portland therapist. But you'll feel hopeful of handling any problems if you take the same active, intelligent role in solving them that you did in your earlier years.

## HEALTH CONCERNS

Ideally, you have been engaging in health-promoting practices over the past years and you're feeling as good now as you did in your twenties and thirties. But unfortunately, many of us don't do all that we should in the way of proper nutrition, exercise, and stress management. Moreover, some of us are genetically predisposed to various illnesses and infirmities. There's no guarantee of lifelong good health for anyone.

Health problems can be hard enough to cope with, but particularly when you work in an emotionally and physically demanding job. Many health care jobs require workers to lift patients or heavy equipment, stand on their feet for most of the day, or walk long distances in the course of a day's work. This strenuous physical activity can be overwhelming for some workers in their later years. In addition, health care jobs can be accompanied by excessive emotional stress, further straining the physical resources.

Health care workers must perform their duties without compromising their own health. Proper utilization of body mechanics is important at any age, but essential for the older worker. Even if you've had no previous history of lower back trouble, you need to take every precaution when lifting or transferring patients and equipment. Work simplification and energy conservation methods can be incorporated into your daily routine, particularly if you have an orthopedic or cardiac condition. Whenever possible, take advantage of techniques and equipment that enable you to perform your job with greater ease and safety.

Some older workers will find themselves unable to adapt their jobs to accommodate their physical limitations. Certain health care jobs can be modified to some extent, but there still will be basic duties and responsibilities that can't be eliminated. There can come a point at which older workers may do patients, other staff, and themselves a disservice by remaining in a position they're no longer capable of performing successfully. If you see this happening to you, don't wait until your health or your job performance deteriorates so that you have no choice but to retire. Speak to your supervisor about your problems and see what, if anything, can be worked out for you. It may be possible, for instance, to reduce the amount of time you're assigned to direct patient care. Some of your younger coworkers may prefer to concentrate on patient care and to leave the bulk of paperwork to you. By restructuring your job to a predominantly sedentary one, it may be possible to continue working productively.

### KEEPING CURRENT

One of the biggest concerns of many older health care workers is how to keep up with current trends and practices. Their professional schooling some 30 to 40 years earlier was quite different than that of recent graduates. It can be difficult for older workers to relate to the current scientific knowledge and technological advances in the health care field. As an occupational therapist explains:

> When I became an occupational therapist (more years ago than I care to reveal), the field was entirely different than it is today. I felt like I was well prepared to practice OT years ago, but it's evolved now into something which feels very foreign to me.
>
> To be perfectly fair, the changes didn't happen overnight. They occurred gradually and, in retrospect, I can see

that they were beneficial both for patients and for the profession itself. But I stubbornly resisted most of the changes, preferring instead to practice "old-fashioned OT." Rather than taking advantage of opportunities to expand my knowledge and skills, I clung to the tried and true. Since some of the new developments were just coming out, there were other therapists in the same boat of not keeping up with what was going on. Little by little, though, most of my colleagues *did* learn and adapted to the changes in our profession.

I suppose I would have had to come to terms with the new developments had I stayed on. Instead, I quit to become a full-time homemaker. I still leafed through professional journals from time to time, but avoided articles on the most current topics and practices. Things like biofeedback, neurodevelopmental therapy, sensory integration, and all those new splinting materials terrified me. I looked for articles on things I could relate to, but there were less and less, until finally, I gave up on it altogether.

Last year, however, personal circumstances forced me to go back to work. I had no choice but to learn all the new techniques and theories. I was determined to do it and I did, but it was damn hard. It was like starting out all over again, learning what amounted to a brand new profession. It would have been a whole lot easier had I kept up with everything that was happening from the beginning. I could have absorbed the new aspects more gradually and it would have been less overwhelming.

Regardless of your age or work history, you need to be committed to do all you can to keep up with the new developments in your field. It can be difficult, stressful, and time-consuming to do this, especially if you're an older worker who feels that suddenly your profession is changing so much that you can barely recognize it. It can be tempting to take the easy way out and convince yourself that you really don't need to learn any new skills or procedures, that a lot of these are just fads that are soon replaced by some other theory. But it's absolutely essential for you to continually upgrade your skills and knowledge if you want to remain a full-fledged member of the health care team.

The easiest way to keep abreast of current developments in your field is to regularly read professional journals and books. If you lack the discipline to sit down and read on your own, form a study group or journal club. Each participant can be assigned an article to present to the group. The atmosphere should be informal, supportive, and encourage free discussion. In addition to the educational aspect of these meetings, there should also be some time allotted for socializing so that members can get to know each other on a personal, rather than just a professional, basis.

More formal learning can take place through workshops and seminars. You can't take advantage of every continuing education opportunity, but if you choose carefully, the ones you do attend can greatly enhance your professional development. Most employers offer paid time off and tuition reimbursement for work-related courses. If yours doesn't, campaign for a liberal educational-leave-and-tuition-payment policy.

You can also consider attending a college course in your field. If the thought of going back to school with all those bright young people is intimidating, remind yourself that you've already proven that you have what it takes. You've shown that you have the brains and the diligence to graduate from your professional curriculum. In addition, you've also got many years of experience behind you, which is something that an eighteen-year-old doesn't have. So don't hesitate to return to school. You can enroll as a regular student or you can audit a class.

Don't overlook younger coworkers as an invaluable source of help in keeping yourself up-to-date. A close relationship with a recent graduate can be mutually beneficial. You can learn a great deal about current trends and practices from your young colleague, and in turn, he or she can utilize you as a learning resource. You may not be well-versed in the latest technological developments, but you do have knowledge and expertise in handling patients that can come only from years of experience. Teaching and advising a younger colleague can be a real ego booster, serving as a reminder that you still have something important to contribute.

## EMPLOYMENT OPPORTUNITIES

At this point in your career, you are less likely to switch jobs as often as you did in the past. Perhaps you'll remain in your present job until you retire. But there is still the possibility that you're currently job-hunting or will be in the near future. You may need to find a new job because your spouse has been transferred; it could be that you're unhappy with the job you're in now. Whatever the reason, looking for a job can be difficult at best. It can be especially trying when you're an older worker.

It's unfair that workers in their fifties and sixties sometimes face discrimination in the job market. There's no basis for this ageism. Most older people are superior workers. Many studies have found that older workers are more reliable, with lower turnover rates and less absences than younger ones. Older employees are typically more resourceful than their junior counterparts since they've had more opportunities to learn to cope with various situations. Older people can also be more patient, tolerant, and compassionate than younger people because they've personally experienced more losses and struggles. Another plus is that older people are relatively free of the personal conflicts distracting those in the early stages of their career; they're less likely to have family or financial problems. Older workers are more apt to have come to terms with themselves and with life in general, freeing their energies for productivity and generating what we call a mature attitude.

Be proud of your maturity. There's no need to apologize for not being twenty years old any more. On the other hand, you don't need to make a point of your age. You're not required by law to give your age on a job application form. It's also not illegal for you to lie about your age; your employer can't take you to court for fraud if it is later discovered that you didn't tell the truth about your age or birthdate.[1] This practice isn't recommended, since it's dishonest and can later backfire on you when it's time to collect your pension. You're better off simply not answering questions about your age. If the question comes up, quietly state that your age has no relevance to your ability to perform the job. Tell your interviewer that you are confident that you can handle the duties and responsibilities that the position entails.

It's against the law to deny a job, promotion, or salary increase because of age. You also can't be fired just before a pension would come due, nor can you be forced into retirement against your will before the age of seventy. If you feel that you're not being hired, promoted, or allowed to continue working because of your age, there are federal labor laws to protect you. To file suit, find a good labor lawyer or go to your local Legal Aid office. This is not a step to be taken lightly, so you'll need to be certain that your age was the sole consideration in your forced retirement or in your not being hired or promoted. Make sure that your work history qualifies you for the job in question. Remember that it's not age discrimination if you're fired because your job performance has truly been unsatisfactory or if you object to adapting to new techniques that have been instituted; or if you're not hired because of a lack of relevant experience or references that attest to your ability to perform the job.

### RETIREMENT PLANNING

Retirement isn't something that you should just allow to happen when you reach a certain age. It requires the same degree of planning and preparation that you put into choosing and developing your career. You should do everything you can to ensure that your retirement will be a positive experience rather than merely the cessation of work.

One of the most important ways that you can prepare for retirement is to develop hobbies and interests outside of work. You may have dreamt for years about what you'd do when you didn't have to work every day. But when it comes time to retire and you're actually faced with 24 unstructured hours each day, you may find that all that free time isn't the blessing you thought it would be. If you don't develop a variety of meaningful leisure activities now, you may well be bored, restless, and frustrated during retirement.

When cultivating leisure interests, keep an open mind. Don't write off any activity too quickly. Hobbies that you never knew anything about or that you never had any interest in may suddenly develop an appeal when work no longer demands 8 or more hours of your day. Analyze what elements you might miss about work and see if you can replace them in your retirement activities. For example, if you're going to miss the close contact with people, get involved with hobby/special-interest/religious/ political organizations where you can mingle with others. If you want to keep up the satisfaction of performing socially useful work, sign up for volunteer work where you can still make a contribution. Express aspects of yourself that were submerged during your career years. If you worked in a highly technical, detail-oriented field, for instance, you may appreciate an outlet for the creativity you were never able to express. Explore creative activities such as sculpture, painting, ceramics, jewelry making, mime, creative writing, or gourmet cooking; you'll eventually be rewarded with the discovery of some hobbies you can pursue more fully when you're retired. One retired health worker looms rugs of his own design. "I used to watch the patients weaving on the loom in the recreation room," he says, "and think, 'I'd love to get my hands on that thing!' "

While exploring leisure interests, also try to develop friendships outside of work. Many people depend on their jobs to provide them with friends and acquaintances for after-hours socializing. But once you retire and are no longer involved with what's going on at the workplace, you may find that you don't have enough in common with your former coworkers for you to have much to say to each other. To make sure that you'll still have an active social life after you retire, begin to form relationships with neighbors, club members, and people you meet at social and community affairs. Accept and reciprocate invitations from people *not* from the job.

Finances are an important aspect of retirement planning. How and where you spend your retirement years will depend on how well you've planned in the years before retirement. To begin planning, you'll need to figure out what you have now, what you'll have when you retire, what you'll need after retirement, and how to get what you need. If doing this seems overwhelming, get a book on financial planning from your library or bookstore. You can also consult a good financial planner/investment advisor/stockbroker. The sooner you establish a plan for saving and investing wisely, the better your financial picture will be when you retire. You'll need to do some work on your own before your visit to the financial planner. Check with your personnel office about pension benefits you'll be entitled to. Also visit your local Social Security office to get an estimate of what your monthly benefits will be when you retire. The financial planner will need this information when figuring out your investment strategy.

Don't panic if your retirement income (pension, Social Security, and investment interest and dividends) is less than what you're earning. Work expenses such as uniforms, books, union and professional association dues, and meals away from home will be eliminated. Transportation costs will be reduced. By the time you retire, your children will probably have finished their education and be on their own, and it is quite possible that your mortgage will be paid off, so you'll no longer have these major expenses. In addition, your investment advisor will probably be able to suggest changes in your assets that could produce more income for you during your retirement years. Also consider developing a moneymaking hobby or skill which would be satisfying on both a personal and financial level.

Your last years of work and your retirement years can be the most rewarding of your entire life. The wisdom, maturity, and experience that you've gained over the years can be used to your advantage. In your work you were dedicated to putting other people's comfort first. Now you're not only allowed to think first of your own satisfaction and enjoyment, you're admired for doing so. People say with respect of a contented retiree: "She (he) has a really nice life." And conveyed in this is optimism for their own eventual retirement. For, working or retired, we always set an active example.

*Chapter 6*

# STRESS AND BURNOUT

As a student and later as a beginning nurse, I found it difficult to understand how any nurse could get burned out. Nursing seemed so exciting and rewarding; how could anyone possibly ever get burnt out on it? I was sure it couldn't happen to me since I had so much energy and commitment to my work.

But after 7 years of psychiatric nursing, I now understand why so many nurses get burnt out. I've been learning about it from personal experience. I may not be as burnt out as some nurses I've seen, but I'm well on my way. I feel tired almost all the time and I've been getting headaches on a daily basis at work. I find myself watching the clock all the time on the job. Although I'm usually very reliable, I can't get myself to work on time any more. Some days I can't force myself to go to work at all.

I'm not proud to admit it, but I don't relate to patients as well as I used to. I don't see them as people any more; now it's just "the manic-depressive in 511" or "the paranoid schizophrenic in 520." I find myself getting annoyed with them and resenting any demands they try to make on me.

When one of them comes to me to talk about a problem, I barely listen. Even worse, I find myself avoiding them as much as I can. I give them their meds, write a few notes, and that's about it. Then I start hating my job even more because it seems like all I do is just hand out pills.

The obvious solution would be to change jobs and go into another field of nursing, but I'm not convinced that it would eliminate the problem entirely. It might help for a while, but I imagine I'd eventually get burnt out again because I know a lot of other nurses in other specialties who are just as burnt out as I am. I've even considered going back to school to study something else, but I don't think I have the energy for it.

—Licensed practical nurse,
Boston

Any occupation which requires its workers to deal closely with other people can be stressful. Teachers, lawyers, prison guards, policemen, and child care workers can all experience an overload of stress. Even workers who perform routine services involving the public, such as waitresses and bus drivers, complain about the stress that their work entails. Because health care workers are especially prone to high levels of stress and severe burnout, it is imperative for them to be alert to the problem, commit themselves to do something about it, and to take action to bring about positive change.

## UNDERSTANDING STRESS AND BURNOUT

No one in our society is immune from stress, nor should they be. Although stress is almost always referred to as a negative factor, it can be a desirable phenomenon. Moderate amounts of stress are a necessary stimulus for growth. Without a sufficient amount of stress, our lives would be stagnant and boring. Too much stress, on the other hand, can be emotionally and physically harmful.

While all people experience some degree of personal or professional stress, not everyone burns out. Some people are naturally able to tolerate high levels of stress for long periods of time. Others experience intense stress but are able to take measures to prevent it from becoming too debilitating. Stress, therefore, is not synonymous with burnout; but it is a necessary precursor to its occurrence.

Burnout is currently a popular concept in professional and popular literature, but it's a phenomenon that's existed for years. The term is often misused by people in all walks of life to denote anything from low levels of stress to career stagnation. Used in its purest sense, burnout can be defined as the total depletion of energy, enthusiasm, and commitment resulting from constant demands on personal resources. As related to health care workers, it can be considered

> . . . the process by which a once-committed health professional becomes ineffective in managing the stress of frequent emotional contact with others in the helping context, experiences exhaustion, and as a result, disengages from patients, colleagues, and the organization.[1]

It's not surprising that burnout is so prevalent among health care workers. The estimate has been calculated that 3 hours on the job as a health professional are equal to 8 hours of work in another type of job.[2] There are certain inherent factors in the nature of health care work that play a major role in conducing burnout. While workers in other fields may also be exposed to some of these causative factors, it's usually not to the degree experienced by a health professional.

Many jobs require their workers to deal closely with the general public. Sales, restaurant, and clerical work all involve a great deal of people contact. But none of these fields necessitates the type of intimate contact that characterizes the majority of health care jobs. Dealing with people in routine, impersonal, and relatively trivial transactions doesn't even begin to approximate the interpersonal demands made on health care workers. Health providers often deal with patients in circumstances that are overwhelming. When a person's well-being is at stake, even small mundane details become crucial. Even if the health care provider is unaware of it at the time, every aspect of the job is pervaded by some degree of stress. The physical closeness to human suffering and distress impinges on the health care worker at a deeper level than anything experienced by workers in other "people jobs." As a respiratory therapist notes:

> Whenever I tell my best friend how stressful my work is, she always lets me know about the stresses of her job. I'm quite sure that selling shoes is no picnic, but I don't see how you could compare her workday with mine. She seems to think that our jobs have equal levels of stress because we have so much contact with people all day long. What she doesn't understand is the difference in the contact. Hers is impersonal and unemotional; not too many people are afraid, uncomfortable, or depressed when trying on shoes. But in my dealings with people, they have all those emotions and more. You can't begin to compare fitting a pair of shoes on someone who's relatively happy and healthy with adjusting a nasal cannula on a critically ill patient who's in a lot of pain and emotional turmoil.

Workers in other fields don't experience the life-and-death pitch of emotions known to health care personnel. In non-health care jobs, workers may have to handle exasperation or frustration, but which is targeted on a material, remediable issue. While customer service personnel, for example, have to deal on a regular basis with irate customers (who can be appeased), health care workers regularly deal with the entire spectrum of emotions in their patients and also in themselves. The anger that an outraged customer might vent in a car dealership can be stressful for the customer service manager. But it's incomparably more stressful for the nurse to encounter the despair of a patient fearing an unfavorable outcome or enduring pain.

Hostility, resentment, frustration, bitterness, and depression are all too well-known to health professionals. Not only are they exposed to these emotions in patients. They themselves enter into some of these feelings. Unless they rigidly distance themselves from their patients, they're bound to feel some anger or frustration when, despite their devoted efforts, some patients don't improve. Health care workers also experience times of triumph. But even these can become stressful. According to one registered nurse:

> When people hear that I work in the labor and delivery room, they immediately think I've got it made. "It must be such *happy* work," they say, and they're right—most of the time. When a delivery goes well and both mother and baby are fine, there's an incredibly upbeat atmosphere. But what people don't realize is that it can be exhausting to deal with such intense highs. It might sound crazy, but all the joy and happiness is sometimes an overload on my system. What makes it especially hard is having to deal with those occasional lows in the midst of all the highs. When something goes wrong and the end result isn't a healthy baby, I'm forced to shift gears and cope with the grief. I often wish I could avoid all those emotional peaks and valleys altogether and find a job where I'd be on emotionally neutral ground.

Another source of stress for health care workers is the *unrelenting* demand for efficiency and accountability. Workers in other jobs are allowed occasional "off days." If they're experiencing family problems or just a general feeling of malaise, a sympathetic boss might lighten their workload on a temporary basis. Many aspects of office work can be shifted onto another employee or delayed for a few days, enabling the troubled employee to slack off for a short while until his or her equilibrium is regained.

This is never the case with health care providers. Health care duties require a 100 percent effort at all times. It doesn't matter if the worker isn't feeling well or is having a marital crisis. Once on duty, all that matters is that that worker provide the very best care possible. Lab workers can't let their stray minds to their marriage breakup; even a relatively small error can alter the test results and then result in improper diagnosis and treatment for the patient in question. A migraine or sinus flareup doesn't allow nursing personnel to take it easy for the rest of their shift. There are too many patients depending on them, patients whose treatment and comfort can't wait until the next day.

In addition to their professional sense of responsibility, health professionals are acutely aware of the legal implications of every action they take. "Accountability" has become a code word for the escalating threat of lawsuits for malpractice and negligence. Although nurses, therapists, and other personnel have little power and authority in comparison to physicians, they're often held *more liable* than the attending physicians when an issue arises.

The lack of autonomy and power can be a significant stress factor for most health care workers. When workers don't feel that they have any real *control* over their work environment, a sense of helplessness and frustration can take hold. Workers feel victimized by a system that doesn't allow them to effect any meaningful changes, so they begin to lose the energy and commitment to try to make an impact on the health care system. The end result is a vicious circle in which it becomes impossible ever to gain any self-determination and to change the status quo.

There are definitely intrinsic rewards for health professionals, but aside from that, the reward system is deficient at best. Most health care organizations don't utilize an efficient and equitable distribution system for rewarding their employees.[3] Paychecks can be insultingly low for many health workers. In some localities, nurses are paid less than garbage collectors and parking meter repairmen. Radiation technologists typically receive lower salaries than unionized factory workers. The problem is further compounded by the lack of financial recognition for seniority. In a large corporation, workers with years of seniority are paid significantly higher salaries than new employees, but in many hospitals, there's only a difference of $2,000 between the annual salaries of beginning nurses and those with 20 years of experience.[4] In addition, there are often variations in the pay scales of health occupations with similar levels of education and responsibilities, and this can seem unfair, as one occupational therapist notes:

> In the hospital I work at, starting salaries for occupational therapists are about 20 percent less than those for physical therapists. The hospital justifies this by saying that they have more trouble hiring PTs. I understand the laws

of supply and demand, but it still seems unfair that someone
with a 4-year degree just like mine who's doing essentially
the same type of work as me is making $5,000 a year more.
Sometimes I wonder if I should do 20 percent less work
than the PTs since the hospital seems to think I'm only worth
80 percent of a PT!

The deficient reward system isn't confined to financial remuneration. There are less tangible rewards, such as recognition,
encouragement, and appreciation. Health care workers are *expected* to do their jobs well; their competent performance is taken
for granted. If their performance is lacking in any way, this will
be pointed out through evaluations, disciplinary action, or ter-
mination; but they're usually not rewarded for excellence.
Whereas productive salespeople can receive a substantial bonus,
promotions, or letters of commendation from the company
president, health professionals are less likely to receive such rewards. Promotional opportunities are limited and recognition
from administration is seldom offered for superior patient care.
Nurses might go well beyond the call of duty in providing comfort
to a patient in need, but they may never know that their efforts
have been noticed and appreciated. Not only are administrative
personnel unlikely to offer any recognition, but patients are
equally unlikely to do so. Patients can't be expected to provide
positive reinforcement; they're usually too worried or uncomfortable to convey great appreciation. Colleagues in other health
care fields would appear to be a source of support and encouragement but, quite often, there's some competition between the
disciplines. Nurses and allied health professionals have long be-
moaned the fact that physicians don't recognize their worth, but
even health care workers themselves can be reluctant to acknowledge the contribution of their peers. According to a physical therapy assistant:

> When I was a student, I was really excited when my
> first patient, a CVA, began to make progress. When the
> patient regained most of her function and was able to return
> home to live independently, I was thrilled. I probably made
> a fool of myself, walking around with a big smile and telling

anyone who would listen that I was so happy that I choose PT for a career since it enabled me to make such a difference in someone's life like that.

What I didn't expect was other people's reactions. An occupational therapist became very defensive and said, "You didn't do it all by yourself, you know. OT had just as much to do with her rehabilitation." The speech therapist said, "I'm tired of PT always trying to take the credit. It was her language improvement that really made the difference." One of the nurses retorted, "Maybe someday you therapists will realize that your work is meaningless unless the patient is medically stable, and we nurses are responsible for that."

I was crushed. I honestly hadn't meant anything by my remark. I wasn't implying that I was solely responsible for the patient's recovery. All I was trying to do was to voice my good feelings about my contribution, but I got shot down by everyone else. I had hoped that my coworkers would share in my happiness, but it didn't seem to work out that way.

The final blow came when a physician who had overheard our conversation said, "What makes any of you think that you really did anything for the patient? Can you prove to me that she wouldn't have recovered on her own without any therapy at all?"

In addition to the stress of dealing with people, there is that of dealing with complex machinery. Technological advances in the health fields have necessitated that most health professionals use highly intricate machines on a regular basis. This can be quite stressful if the machines aren't understood completely or if workers feel that they have to rely too much on the machines and not enough on themselves for the performance of their duties. Many health professionals choose a career in health care because they wanted to work with *people,* but are now finding that they're working more with *machines.*

Most hospitals and other health facilities chronically suffer from staffing problems. This adds significant stress to the work lives of many health care personnel, since overtime, work overloads, and "floating coverage" are the inevitable results. Having to work many consecutive days without any time off or having to accept overtime on a regular basis can contribute to burnout. Being "on call" or working on an as-needed basis can be draining since expected days off may never materialize. Alternating shift work can be physically taxing, as can placement in units or departments other than the one to which the worker is regularly assigned. When staff shortages force employees to work in unfamiliar surroundings, the tension of having to become acclimated to different patients, personnel, and procedures is added to the usual stresses encountered in their typical work days. Many health care workers have unpredictable workloads in which they have to handle both routine tasks and emergencies as they arise. Having to suddenly shift gears from the methodical pace of paperwork ("I've got a nice rhythm going") and other job duties to the high-key physical and emotional demands required in emergency situations can take its toll on health care workers.

Yet another source of stress is the ever-increasing paperwork requirements. Health personnel often feel frustrated when they find themselves spending more time on paperwork and other bureaucratic necessities than on actual patient care. Almost without exception, health care workers go into the field to work with people, not to fill out forms, and may become disillusioned when their careers turn out to be more writing and less action than they had expected.

The physical structure of the work environment can have an impact on the health professional's experience.[5] Many units have inadequate space for the number of patients, personnel, and supplies that need to be accommodated. Overcrowding can make it difficult for workers to perform their duties efficiently. Lighting and ventilation can be poor. Overstimulation of the olfactory (via medicinal smells, patients' body odors, cleaning solutions, food, flowers, and excrement) and the auditory senses (from patients' moans, sobs of family members, respirators, P.A. system) is also wearing.

Regardless of the field they're in, workers can't expect stress-free work environments and job duties. Stress is a fact of life for almost everyone. But health care workers are continually exposed to an inordinate amount. While any health care worker can experience burnout, but certain workers may be especially prone.

Maslach, a psychologist regarded as one of the foremost authorities on the subject, notes that young single females probably have the greatest proclivity for burning out.[6] Younger people are more likely to burn out because they tend to be highly idealistic, seeking perfection in a flawed world. When their unrealistic expectations aren't met, they become disillusioned. Older people have a more balanced and tolerant approach. People with families experience less burnout because they divide their emotional energies between work and their spouses and children. Single people are more apt to suffer from burnout because they may have to rely exclusively on work to satisfy their emotional needs. Females are more likely to experience emotional exhaustion, since women have typically been expected to be more nurturant and sensitive to other people's feelings than men.

Maslach also notes that certain personality characteristics can be associated with an increased tendency towards burnout.[7] People who are submissive and unassertive in dealing with people may burn out quickly since they have difficulty setting limits in a helping relationship. Lack of negotiating skills prevents these health care workers from developing mutually profitable relationships with staff and patients; quite often, they may be taken advantage of by their coworkers and even their patients. A lack of self-confidence can be stressful in itself since the health care worker may never feel fully capable of performing the necessary duties, leading to a chronic feeling of being overwhelmed. A tendency towards perfectionism can contribute to burnout, since these individuals may set unattainable standards for themselves and others. Health care workers who empathize to an excessive degree with their patients are apt to experience burnout because of the emotional overload. Type A personalities are extremely vulnerable. So are professionals who continually push themselves to do more and more, denying any limits to their emotional and physical resources. Health care workers who have difficulty establishing close relationships with their colleagues or to use supportive networks are more likely to burn out, since isolation exacerbates this condition.

No health field or setting is immune from burnout. When thinking about likely situations for its onset, a field like O.R. nursing immediately comes to mind. But any field can be a conducive setting. Psychiatric nursing may use less sophisticated equipment and the pace may be slower than that in the O.R., but it has its own unique stress factors such as the potential for patients in severe mental distress.

Geriatric nursing can be a field in which many workers experience burnout since geriatric facilities are usually understaffed. Nurses may then be responsible for the acts of minimally trained aides or orderlies.[8] The low prestige associated with geriatric nursing is another contributor to burnout, since it can impair self-esteem. Working with acute patients can be stressful since there may not be enough time to get to know patients as people or to see meaningful improvement; but it can be equally stressful to work with chronic patients where one cannot detect any progress. Health occupations with high people-contact are more likely to promote burnout, but any health field has its own demands and pressures that can be responsible.

Burnout does not happen overnight. It occurs gradually and in several stages. All burnt-out workers initially began their careers with a great deal of enthusiasm. High hopes and seemingly unlimited energy are prevalent during this "honeymoon period."[9] Workers may feel that the job is everything in life; nothing else really matters. There is a tendency to work extra hours and assume additional responsibilities, all on a voluntary basis. They may feel extremely close to patients, completely identifying and empathizing with them. Workers in the first stage are sincere in their desires to do well in their work; but even the most dedicated worker has only so much energy to give before it's depleted. When this happens, workers can experience a vague feeling of loss as they realize subconsciously that the honeymoon is over. There can still be surges of energy, but bouts of fatigue follow. The job may no longer be as engrossing. The worker is still capable of performing, but can be inefficient at times, and may have trouble keeping up with necessary duties.

As time goes on, dissatisfaction with the job may deepen if energy continues to be depleted without being recharged. Symptoms become chronic. The worker becomes aware that something is happening to him, or to her. Just the thought of going to work can be exhausting. The worker begins to question his own effectiveness in doing the job, and the value of the job itself.

As the condition continues, the apathy stage develops as a defense mechanism against the frustration experienced in the job. The worker doesn't necessarily quit, but decides that it's "just a job." The job is necessary for economic survival, but it doesn't provide any personal satisfaction. The worker never invites any new challenges, tries to avoid patients as much as possible, and puts in only the minimum time. Workers in this stage assume a cynical, dehumanized, negative attitude towards patients, and then feel alienated from *themselves* for feeling this way.

With appropriate intervention, recovery is possible in any of the preceding stages. In the final stage of terminal burnout, the outlook is poor. Workers in this stage are completely soured on themselves and on people. Job performance is minimal at best.

## RECOGNIZING THE SYMPTOMS OF BURNOUT

As Edelwich and Brodsky note:

> One cannot smooth out the surf, but one can ride the waves—if one sees them coming.[10]

Therefore, it is important for all health care workers to be aware of the signs of stress and burnout. The problem cannot be treated until it is recognized. One or two of the following symptoms[11] does not automatically indicate burnout, but a number of them on a chronic basis may be indicative of a real problem.

*Physical*

    Fatigue
    Sleeping disorders (too much or too little sleep)
    Weight loss or gain
    Headaches

Backaches
Stomach ailments
Shortness of breath
Nausea
Frequent or lingering colds
Frequent injuries

*Psychological*

Self-doubt
Frustration
Cynicism
Disillusionment
Resentment
Anxiety
Apathy
Boredom
Anger
Resignation
Moodiness
Irritability
Lack of enthusiasm

*Behavioral*

Avoidance of patients (including limited eye contact and physical distancing from patient)
Dehumanization of patients, seeing just their illnesses or focusing on one system rather than the total patient)
Absenteeism
Taking extended meal times and breaks
"Going by the book" rather than trying innovative new techniques and ideas
Drug/alcohol/cigarette abuse

Increased concern with own well-being and less about the
welfare of others

Isolation from colleagues

Stereotyping patients

Ridiculing patients

Clock-watching

Hyperactivity or hypoactivity

Increased concern with technical (rather than interpersonal)
aspects of the job

Increased problems at home

Patronizing patients

Tardiness

Inattention to details

Poorly charted notes and observations

Frequent complaining about job

## MAKING A COMMITMENT TO SOLVING THE PROBLEM

Burnout doesn't go away on its own. Without intervention,
it continues until there's nothing left to burn out and there's
virtually no hope for recovery. The worker's performance suffers
dramatically, often to the point where patients are receiving such
poor care that their health or lives are endangered. The worker
may decide that quitting is the only alternative or may be ter-
minated by the employer. Even if the worker is able to function
marginally well enough to continue working, work becomes an
ordeal to dread and endure.

Unfortunately, workers in the more advanced stages of
burnout aren't in a position where they can easily reverse the
process. Because their emotional and physical resources are so
drained, it can be impossible to exert the effort to do anything
about the crisis. The apathy characteristic of burnout prevents
the worker from actively seeking solutions and taking the appropriate measures; the cynicism may even lead the burnt-out
worker to disparage any real hope for improvement.

But, with the exception of the relatively small percentage of cases with the most advanced, irreversible stage of burnout, there *are* solutions. With determination, workers will find that there are things they can do to alleviate the problem and even reverse it.

Burnt-out workers get into a rut and become overwhelmed by a sense of futility. When asked whether they're doing anything to counteract this, they are likely to respond, "Why bother?" "What can you do?" But if you're experiencing burnout, you need to realize that there definitely are some reasons why you should bother to do something to prevent and diminish burnout:

1. *Deep down, you're still hooked on the idea of working in health care.*

There's still a commitment to your profession and an idealism about what you're doing. It may have diminished over the years and sometimes it may seem like it's not there at all, but when you hear your profession come under fire, you react with, "Hey, wait a minute!" When the subject comes up on TV or in the press, you feel a little jab, like hearing of an old boy or girlfriend. Then you realize that although it can be boring, frustrating, and exhausting, when the chips are down, you're still loyal to the belief that there's some worth in what you're doing.

According to a medical social worker:

> After 8 years, I began to burn out on my job. There were just so many clients to deal with and so many problems to handle that I became exhausted. I felt like I was going around in circles. As soon as I had solved one client's problems, there were 10 more waiting to take his or her place. I was burning out fast and ready to give up on social work.
>
> I was seriously thinking of quitting, but my employer arranged for me to go to a social work conference. I couldn't have cared less about it; I only went as an escape from work. But while I was there, I found myself really enjoying the conference. I realized that I was becoming excited about social work again. The conference seemed to reignite a spark in me that had lain dormant for a long time. I discovered that, even with all its problems, I still believed in social work and its power to make a difference in people's lives.

2. *The effects of your job burnout are spilling into every part of your life.*

Even if you could learn to live with the emotional and physical consequences of burnout while you're at work, you want to be able to enjoy your nonworking hours. When the effects of burnout become so pervasive as to interfere with the quality of your personal life, it is imperative to take corrective steps. As an emergency medical technician says:

> I always thought it was a sign of weakness to admit to having problems. When people would ask me how I managed to cope with such a stressful job, I would try to minimize the impact the work was having on me. "You get used to it," I'd say. But in reality, you never do. The pace, the pressure, the responsibilities can be overwhelming. I thought the best way to deal with it was not to deal with it at all. I tried to ignore the warning signs as long as I could, but eventually I couldn't deny it any longer: I was really burnt out.
>
> I still wasn't ready to do anything about it. I decided that I'd just learn to live with it while I was working and then I could forget about it when I got home. But it didn't work that way. Pretty soon, I discovered that burnout isn't something you simply leave behind when your shift is over. It invades every aspect of your life. My relationship with my wife and kids suffered. I lost interest in my hobbies. Finally, when one of the other EMTs confided in me about how his burnout had ultimately led to the destruction of his marriage, I realized that I was going to have to do something about my problem. I didn't want to see my whole life go down the drain because I hadn't done anything to help myself.

3. *You're making more money in your health care job than you would if you started doing something else.*

Working in nursing or allied health won't make you rich, but thankfully, many employers have started to pay decent salaries. If you've been working for a while, you may finally be earning a wage you can live on. Switching career fields might mean a cut in salary for you. For some people, this can be a small price to pay; they'd gladly learn to live on less money to be able to begin a new career. Other people may not be willing or able to sacrifice part of their salary. As a pharmacist explains:

> I've really burnt out on pharmacy and I'd love to quit. Anything would be better than filling another prescription. Lately I've become interested in public relations and marketing. I think those fields would be very interesting to work in. But there's no way I could ever change careers. It's possible to make a lot of money in PR, but not when you first start out. As a beginner with no experience, I'd be making less than half of what I'm making now. As a single mother raising two kids, I can't afford to take a cut in pay like that. I'm just going to have to stay in pharmacy and make the best of it.

4. *You're not sure of what you'd rather do as an alternative to a health care career.*

Paid work is a necessity for most of us. If you have to work but aren't happy in the health care field, the obvious solution would be a career change. But knowing that you'd like to switch your line of work doesn't necessarily mean that you know exactly what it is that you'd prefer. Until you discover what you would like to do with the rest of your work life and can pursue it, you'll probably need to remain in your health care job. If this is so, you need to treat your burnout so that you can effectively function in your job until you're able to make the switch. As a former speech pathologist notes:

> I burned out after almost 10 years of working in speech therapy. I knew that I had to get out of the field; I couldn't continue like that for 30 more years. But I had no idea of what I wanted to do instead. I couldn't quit my job to spend 6 months trying to discover what I wanted to go into. So I had no choice but to continue working in speech until I found something else. I was forced to do something about my burnout so I could remain on the job and support myself until I worked things out. While I was fortunate enough to

hook up with a really good employment agency that found me a terrific sales position within a few months, I never could have done it without continuing my employment as a speech therapist.

## TAKING ACTION TO COPE WITH STRESS AND BURNOUT

As has been emphasized, stress goes with the health care territory and can't ever be eliminated entirely. But the stress experience is different for each individual and consequently, so is his manner of coping with it. Veninga and Spradley[12] note that there are five dominant coping styles:

1. *Loyal servants*
   Passive compliance is the major operating mode of individuals in this category. They see themselves merely as hired hands whose function is simply to follow orders and do work as assigned.
2. *Angry prisoners*
   Individuals with this coping style tend to use passive resistance. They feel that they don't have any control over their jobs but they balk at yielding compliantly to the demands and stresses that the jobs impose on them. While they don't feel that they're in a position to facilitate any changes, they deeply resent the status quo and rebel against it in subtle ways.
3. *Stress fugitives*
   The trademark of this coping style is avoidance tactics. Individuals in this category try to escape work stress by running away from it. They attempt to avoid the more difficult assignments by procrastinating and even actually neglecting their responsibilities. When stress becomes impossible to escape, they run to a new job.
4. *Job reformers*
   These individuals focus their energy on a crusade for change. Laying all the blame for their stress on the job itself, they try to make their work settings conform to their image of the ideal situation.

5.  *Stress managers*
    Individuals with this coping style strive to identify and
    control stress. Not wanting to ignore or run away from
    it, they analyze the factors that are responsible for their
    stress and develop strategies to reduce or at least main-
    tain the stress to a manageable level.

The following pages offer a variety of stress interventions.
Most of them fall within the coping style used by stress managers,
requiring direct action to diminish or control the stress. A few
(i.e., time off) could be considered to fall under the stress fugitive
category, while others (i.e., changing aspects of the job) are those
utilized by job reformers. None of the suggested interventions
will totally eliminate the stresses of a health care job. In reality,
there are no quick and easy solutions to the occupational battle
fatigue experienced by nursing and allied health personnel. But
with improved coping methods, you can *tolerate* stress, and *prevent*
burnout.

## Restructuring the job

Although the duties and responsibilities of most health care
jobs are quite well-defined, there is always margin for change.
The basic job description can't be changed, but certain aspects
of the job can be modified to reduce stress. Even one or two
small changes can have a positive effect in relieving stress and
burnout. Since the atmosphere and requirements of jobs in the
various health care fields and facilities vary enormously, specific
interventions cannot be suggested, but the following general
strategies may be applied to your unique situation.

Because time is one commodity which busy health professionals never seem to have enough of, time management is crucial. By utilizing the limited time you have available in the most
effective way possible, you'll reduce the pressure and feel that
you've accomplished more. The ultimate goal of time management is to work *smarter,* not *harder.* For example, try to consolidate
tasks whenever possible. Some tasks can be combined, saving you
from having to retrace your steps later and thus conserving both
time and energy. This does not mean, however, that you should

do *two things at once*—i.e., charting while talking on the phone or talking to visitors. Doing two things at once (when each legitimately demands your exclusive attention) places an overload on your system. It can also lead to mistakes, which further adds to your stress and costs you additional time because you have to redo what was wrong.

One of the most important time management techniques is knowing how to utilize your prime time. If you can schedule your most demanding activities for that time when you have peak energy, you'll perform this work most efficiently. Don't try to ignore your biorhythms and keep on "automatic drive" all day long. Acknowledge your energy highs and lows, and their influence on your productivity. If patient care is the most demanding aspect of your job and you function best in the morning, save paperwork or reading professional journals and other more passive and sedentary routines for later in the day when your energy ebbs.

Whenever possible, make a schedule of necessary activities when you begin work each day. Try to separate low-priority or nonproductive activities from the ones that are absolutely necessary or most important. The idea is not to establish a rigid schedule that you follow inflexibly, but to put you in control of your workday rather than at the mercy of your work demands.

In some cases, the actual hours of job duty can be restructured. Shift work may always be a necessary aspect of many health care jobs, but employers are beginning to show willingness to allow more flexibility in scheduling work hours. Whenever possible, try to work the type of schedule that fits your own biorhythms and life-style. Part-time, flex-time, time-sharing, mornings, evenings, and 4-day work weeks can be options to the standard 9 to 5/8 to 4/7 to 3 workdays five times a week.

Scheduled off-duty hours should be as important to you as your on-duty hours. Be protective towards your time off. Make sure you're getting enough of it and in the way that makes you most comfortable. If you find you need 2 full days off to really unwind but you're all too often scheduled for only 1 day off at a time, speak up. Your supervisor may not be thrilled about revising the schedule, but you need to do what's best for you. Some health care workers also need to work towards changing their on-call status. Although they're technically off duty when on call, the knowledge that their free time could be suddenly interrupted by a phone call or a beeper message can prevent these workers from truly relaxing and enjoying their time off. If you find yourself in this group, work with administration to develop a better plan, one that will ensure adequate coverage while providing you with quality leisure time.

Also, along this vein, learn to be assertive in saying no to overtime. You didn't take an oath to work 50- or 60-hour weeks when you became a health care professional. All you probably committed yourself to was a 40-hour week when you agreed to accept your current job. Working a 40-hour week in health care can be stressful enough, but working 10 to 20 hours beyond that can definitely lead to burnout. It's true that your place of employment may be short-handed and needs your help desperately, but *you* may need the time off equally desperately. If you're going to avoid burnout, it's essential for you to have sufficient time away from work to balance your personal and professional lives. It falls upon your employer, not you, to adequately staff the facility. Feel free to decline overtime—and do it without guilt.

Almost every school system offers sabbaticals to its teachers, but sabbaticals are generally nonexistent in health care. Push for reforms in this area. An extended period of time off in which a few employees are freed from their regular job duties can be utilized as effectively by health care workers as it is by educators. Whether the sabbatical is 1 month or 1 year, getting out of the daily rut can be refreshing and invigorating. Constructive use of such time could include learning new skills, traveling to study other programs, preparing grant proposals, or developing new programs. This can actually be more meaningful than a vacation in which the employee is away from the demands of work but comes back to find that nothing is changed and that work is as stressful as ever. With the knowledge or skills gained from a sabbatical, workers can restructure their jobs to make them more interesting, challenging, efficient, and ultimately, less stressful.

Similarly, try to attend a few workshops or conferences each year. In addition to altering your daily grind for a day or two, you may be able to pick up new skills, network, or develop improved coping abilities to bring back to your job. It's unrealistic, however, to expect any workshop to solve all your work-related problems. If you can make or renew a contact to enlarge your professional support network or acquire just one small piece of new information, the workshop will have been worthwhile. If all it does is give you something to look forward to for a few weeks— you should make sure you *always* have something to look forward to—or affords you a temporary escape from a stress-filled environment, that's also worthwhile. Just make sure that your expectations for a workshop are realistic. Expecting too much can result in more harm than good. As a registered nurse relates:

> I was really excited about attending a particular workshop a few months ago. It sounded terrific and I was sure that I'd learn a lot. Even more than that, I was depending upon it to revive me professionally. I had been feeling bored and stagnant at work; I needed this to get my professional juices flowing again. I was convinced that things would be better once I attended the seminar.
>
> As it turned out, the workshop was every bit as good as I had hoped. The instructors were excellent and I learned a great deal in just 3 days. I returned to work with my morale and energy level boosted but this "workshop high" soon faded after a couple of days. My coworkers weren't able to share my newfound enthusiasm since they hadn't attended the workshop. And things were exactly the way they were before I left. I soon discovered that the workshop had only been a temporary "fix." In fact, it made things worse because it had given me such high hopes. When I saw that my expectations weren't going to be met, I became very disillusioned.

Health care workers tend not to take full advantage of their meal and break times. All too often, they never seem to take the full time allotted to them. Even if they do take their entire scheduled break, they're apt to misuse it. Eating a quick lunch or dinner in the unit lounge is hardly a break since you really haven't changed your surroundings. Likewise, meals in hospital cafeterias tend to be less than relaxing. The food itself isn't the major culprit; it's the atmosphere. Being around a large number of other employees who are equally rushed and under their own stresses isn't conducive to unwinding. The auditory bombardment of pages over the P.A. system and beepers going off is combined with a great deal of job-centered conversation, never allowing you to escape from health care for even 30 minutes.

In order to minimize your stresses and function better when you return to work, make the most of your breaks. Don't use them for doing chores or making phone calls. Indulge yourself by doing something fun or at least something that totally removes you from the demands of work. Some health care workers find relief from such things as:

> Avoiding the hospital cafeteria whenever possible. Meals and snacks can be brought from home and enjoyed outdoors when weather permits. Local restaurants offer another alternative, provided they're not too popular with your coworkers. If a great many of your fellow workers frequent a particular outside restaurant, it becomes nothing more than an extension of the employee's cafeteria.
>
> Tune out everything by stretching out in the lounge and listening to music on headphones.
>
> Learn self-hypnosis for relaxation.
>
> Psychologists can usually teach you how to hypnotize yourself in a couple of sessions.
>
> Leaf through travel brochures of exotic places.
>
> Plan your next vacation.
>
> Take a mental trip to the ocean, mountains, or any other place you find relaxing.
>
> If your imagination is a little rusty, a relaxation tape can help you get in the mood.
>
> Exercise.
>
> Many health facilities are starting fitness programs for their employees. If your place of work doesn't have such a program, become instrumental in starting one.
>
> Use the hospital chapel.
>
> Even if you're not religious, it can still be an ideal place for reflection and meditation.

Use your breaks to learn something new. Possibilities include:
1. learning a foreign language.
2. reading about a period of history that you find fascinating (i.e., ancient Egypt or the United States in the 1920s).
3. learning a craft, such as knitting, macrame, needlepoint, weaving, sculpture, stained glass, wood carving, cartooning, calligraphy, origami.

Whenever possible, vary your work routine. Even if you can only change relatively small aspects of the job, it will help to reduce stress by giving you a sense of *control* over your work. You probably won't be able to eliminate any of your duties, but you can adjust the *pace* and the *order* in which you complete certain tasks. By adjusting your routine, you can break up the monotony of doing things the same way day after day. You'll also like your job better because you'll have structured it to suit yourself. For example, a nurse can decide which patients to see first, thus allowing him or her to spend some extra time with certain patients.

Try to get some relief from direct care. The more hours of direct, unrelieved contact with people, the greater the risk that a worker will burn out.[13] If your job involves 8 hours of continuous direct care, talk with your coworkers and supervisors to see if jobs couldn't be restructured so that a small portion of every worker's day could be spent away from direct patient care. Even half an hour of relief from the stress of working with patients could be helpful.

To enable health care workers to get some time off from direct patient contact, work would need to be divided up so that everyone does varied tasks, including some administrative duties. This can make the workday less boring and draining for everyone concerned. It also exposes the staff to administrative concerns, helping them to develop an appreciation for the demands placed on their superiors. For workers who eventually would like an administrative job, the opportunity to gain some experience in this area can be very appealing. However, it should be noted that dividing up jobs between several people can lead to confusion, conflict, waste, and inefficiency.[14] Job division must be done very carefully to ensure that it is allocated fairly and efficiently.

If you wait passively for good things to happen, they may never materialize. *Make* them happen in your job, even if only in small ways. One of the best means of doing this in health care is to make the most of the human contact that's intrinsic to your job. Instead of getting caught up in the technical spects of your job, try to really connect with the people you come into contact with. The demands and structure of many health care jobs prohibit lengthy interaction with patients, but even a few minutes of contact can be meaningful for both the health care worker and patient. The brief time spent with a patient can be enhanced if the health care worker makes a conscientious effort to relate to the patient as a human being. A good example of this is provided by a venipuncturist who relates:

> I was starting to get really burnt out on my job. It seemed like all it had boiled down to was just running in and out of patients' rooms to draw blood. Not only did I feel bored and unchallenged, but I was also frustrated by the limited contact I did have with the patients. It had become very depersonalized; I had lost sight of the patients as human beings and was seeing them just as veins that I had to get a sample from. And it seemed that the patients weren't really seeing *me;* all I was to them was an intruder in a white uniform who was going to poke at their arms.
>
> I didn't like the way things were going, so I began to look for ways to make the job better. I decided to take the time to talk with each patient for a couple of minutes before I did anything else. I'll always look around their rooms now for something to talk to them about. I make a game of getting clues from the room about what their interests might be. Magazines, books, and personal articles can suggest some interests of that patient. I'll try to compliment them about something, be it a floral arrangement or a robe hanging up on the closet door. Humor can really break the ice, particularly when I poke fun at my job by saying things like "I'm your friendly neighborhood vampire and I've come to take your blood."

Taking the time to relate to each patient I come into contact with has made a big difference in my job. It's not so boring anymore; in fact, it can be quite a challenge to find things to talk about with some patients. It's given me a lot more poise and has improved my self-esteem since patients are now relating more favorably to me. It may take a few extra minutes, but it's been well worth it.

Do whatever you can to convince the higher-ups to allow you and your coworkers to have some input into policy decisions that affect your jobs. Since a perceived lack of autonomy can contribute to burnout, a preventive is being involved in the decision-making process regarding things that affect you and your work on a daily basis. Take advantage of every opportunity to voice your concerns and make your opinion count.

The following sections deal with suggestions for coping with the stresses of a health care job. Every health professional needs to learn intrapersonal and interpersonal strategies for dealing with stress. But it is important to try to push for organizational changes as well. The solution is not just to learn to cope with a stressful job but, as much as possible, to make the job less stressful to begin with. Organizational change might not come easily, but organizations are forced to be receptive to new ideas when the status quo gets costly. Poor employee performance and high rates of turnover and absenteeism will encourage even the largest and most traditional institutions to make some changes. Be persistent in trying to restructure your job to make it less stressful; eventually it will pay off.

### Interpersonal strategies

It has been noted that dealing with people (and patients in particular) can be extremely stressful. The emotional demands of working closely with the sick can never be eliminated entirely, but it is possible to reduce some of the stresses that accompany most health care jobs.

Patients.    Developing an attitude of *"detached concern"* can be one of the most helpful strategies for making your work less emotionally draining. By trying to strike a balance between closeness and distance, you can still be helpful to your patients while reducing the wear and tear on your emotions. Detached concern has long been the professional ideal of physicians who understand that they need to develop a certain objectivity and distance without ceasing to care about their patients. Because of this attitude of detached concern (as well as other factors such as their financial renumeration and autonomy), physicians are less prone to burnout than nursing and allied health personnel.

Nurses and allied health professionals take pride in their ability to empathize with their patients, seeing this characteristic as instrinsic to the helping relationship. But this constant empathizing is severely draining and tends to result in burnout. It is far more advantageous to both professional and patient to empathize on a *cognitive* rather than on an emotional level. *Understanding* a person's problems is not the same as vicariously *experiencing* them. Try to see things from your patient's perspective, but avoid feeling someone else's emotions. As Maslach points out,[15] the helping professional should have the attitude of "I see where you're coming from, but your pain is not going to be mine."

Keep in mind that although your patients need you (and you may need to be needed), you can't be completely responsible for them. You're only responsible for an aspect of each patient's care, within a structured time period. You can't be responsible for everything in his or her life. As an occupational therapist relates:

> I went into O.T. because I felt it was concerned with the whole person. That philosophy really appealed to me since I was determined to help all my patients in a holistic way. As far as I was concerned, a good occupational therapist wasn't concerned with just the patient's motor function and daily living skills; every facet of that patient's life was important. No detail seemed too trivial or irrelevant to deal with. It wasn't just enough to teach a stroke patient how to cook—I worried about how they'd get groceries once they were discharged. It was something a social worker could have done, but I wanted to be involved in every aspect of

my patients' lives. Even when patients were discharged, I
was still involved with them. Eventually I found that I was
concerning myself with patients' financial problems and
family troubles to the point that I didn't have a lot of time
or energy left for anything else. I was neglecting some patients and not focusing on what was uniquely O.T. For the
sake of all my patients as well as to relieve the pressure I
felt myself under, I became more realistic about my role as
a health care provider.

The nature of health care necessitates that workers be concerned with other people's problems. Health care providers are
apt to focus on the negative aspects of their patients. Patients
are seen in terms of dysfunction, disability, illness, poor health
practices, and undesirable personality characteristics. This neg-
ativity can lead to cynicism, disinterest in patients, and increasing
burnout. Striving to find something *positive* about each patient
you work with will help counteract this tendency. If you can
manage to see each one in a favorable light, you'll feel better
about yourself and the work you do. If each patient is seen as
worthwhile and important, then working with them will be viewed
in the same way.

Assertiveness can go a long way in reducing stress. If limits
aren't set in a helping relationship, the emotional demands can
be overwhelming for the helper. Manipulative or demanding
patients can drain the already limited physical and emotional
resources of the health care worker. Keep in mind that it's not
your job to grant every wish or request a patient may have. To
do so would be professionally and personally self-destructive.
Your patients may want things that are not appropriate for their
health needs, go against rules and regulations, or demand more
time and energy than you can spare. Don't be afraid to say no,
don't evade it by saying, "I'll be back," and don't feel guilty about
doing this. If you find it difficult to be assertive, read one of the
many excellent books written on the subject or enroll in an assertiveness training course.

Improving your interpersonal skills will make it easier for
you to deal with people and, consequently, to experience less
stress. Feedback from patients can help you determine what

you're doing right and what you're doing wrong. Unfortunately, patients often neglect to let you know how you're doing. When they do provide feedback, it's more likely to be critical than complimentary. Everyone needs to receive positive strokes, so solicit good feedback if it doesn't occur spontaneously. You can do this by asking your patients to let you know if what you're doing is helpful or to tell you what they like about your work in addition to what they dislike.

*Colleagues.*   Your fellow workers can be either another source of stress or a means of obtaining emotional support and help. Peers can provide comfort, advice, and backing that may be unobtainable from even your closest friends and family. Since they experience similar job demands, your coworkers are uniquely qualified to understand your stresses and help you cope with them.

Try to cultivate a positive relationship with all your coworkers in order to build as large a supportive network as possible. Avoid seeing your peers as competitors. Since there is strength in numbers, health care workers will benefit from a combined cooperative effort. It is counterproductive to put up walls between potential allies. Rather than looking upon workers in other health care fields as rivals for power or prestige, try to add these workers to your support network.

It is quite common for a health care worker to feel that no one else suffers from burnout. The tendency for coworkers to hide their feelings and not discuss them leads each one to mistakenly believe that his or her situation is unique. The individual then sees his or her reactions as being atypical or inappropriate. According to a registered nurse:

> When I first started working, I quickly discovered that I had trouble dealing with some of the stresses I encountered everyday. Patients dying, people suffering, the demands on my energy and emotions all were harder to handle than I thought they would be. What made things especially rough was that I was convinced that I was the only nurse who had trouble handling it. The other nurses seemed so professional, efficient, and in control; it didn't seem possible that

they could be going through the same thing I was. There had to be something wrong with me if I couldn't handle it. I wasn't sure if it was my lack of experience or possibly some sort of innate character flaw that meant I really shouldn't be in nursing, but I felt it was my fault if I found it difficult to cope with the emotional strains of nursing. I didn't dare speak to any of the other nurses. They seemed to be doing fine and wouldn't be able to relate to my problems. It would only make things worse if they knew what I was going through.

When a stress management workshop was advertised in a nearby city, I immediately signed up for it but I didn't let any of my coworkers know. If I told them about the workshop, they'd know I was burning out. So I kept it a secret and went there on my own. Imagine my surprise when I saw a couple dozen nurses from my hospital there! I couldn't understand what they were doing there; they certainly didn't seem to have any trouble coping with stress. But during the course of the workshop, all of us opened up and talked about our feelings. It was hard for me to believe, but all my colleagues who I thought had it so together really didn't. They were experiencing the same frustrations and anxieties that I was. And they felt that they needed to learn to handle it better.

We all learned a lot at that workshop, but one of the most important things I learned was that it's important to share your feelings. By assuming that I was the only one experiencing negative emotions and refusing to talk with anyone about it, I only added to my problems. Things would have had been a whole lot better from the beginning if I had taken a chance and opened up with some of the people I worked with.

Do whatever you can to get in touch with your colleagues. Take advantage of informal opportunities like lunch breaks or off-hour socializing. But also try to establish a more formalized peer support system. Work towards initiating group sessions that occur on a regular basis. These groups work best when conducted by a leader who can provide structure and direction. Since people may feel inhibited if their bosses are there, it may not be appropriate to include supervisors or administrators. Instead, these groups should be reserved for colleagues who are willing to be open, vulnerable, and supportive. There should be an atmosphere of trust and cooperation, leading group members to feel free to discuss their problems and work on solutions.

While some health care workers may find it beneficial to let off steam in informal settings like the staff lounge, it should be noted that these "bitch sessions" usually don't lead anywhere. People may feel better once they've released pent-up feelings, but this is only a temporary relief. Within a short time, workers again experience the same stress reaction because *nothing has changed.* It is far preferable to have a true support group in which members contribute new insights on how to do things better.

Also look toward unions or professional societies for help in the battle against burnout. When people join forces and act as a unified group, they have a greater chance of effecting the kind of changes that will reduce stressful working conditions. If one person complains, the complaint is turned back against the complainer. The attitude of the supervisor or the institution becomes negative toward that individual: "Something must be wrong with *you;* no one else is complaining." But when a *group* of people complain or try to lobby for needed changes, attention is forced away from the individual and focused instead on what is going wrong with the *situation.*[16]

### Personal coping

Since it will never be possible to completely eliminate stress from health care jobs, it is imperative that health care workers learn to cope with it. Stressful professions need stress-tolerant people to function within them.[17] The maintenance of your physical and mental health is essential to ensure adequate job performance as well as a satisfying personal life. The following interventions should prove to be helpful for reducing stress and preventing burnout.

Cultivating *self-awareness* is one of the most important steps that a health care worker can take to prevent burnout. You need to pinpoint exactly what it is that you find stressful and to recognize the symptoms you typically experience. Without this information, you won't be able to develop a strategic plan to combat them. Begin by keeping a daily log to discover *patterns* of emotional stress. Whenever you experience a physical sign (i.e., headache or muscle tension) record the time of day that it occurred and what you were doing at the time. Also note how you attempted to cope with it. After recording this information for a 2 to 4 week period, you should be able to analyze it to ascertain some of the factors causing your stress, and how you try to deal with it. You may find, for example, that you tend to feel pressured during the middle of the morning and attempt to relieve it by grabbing a candy bar, but the cause of your discomfort may actually be low blood sugar rather than what you usually do at mid-morning. You may see that you experience more tension working with older people, possibly because you're having trouble dealing with your own aging parents. From this analysis, you can start to choose the coping techniques that will be right for you in specific situations.

Whatever the cause of your stress and your mechanisms for coping with it, be careful not to blame yourself. Don't feel that something is wrong with you or that you're a failure because you have difficulty dealing with stress. Negative thoughts will only add to it. It's important to talk positively to yourself. Do whatever it takes to remind yourself that, regardless of whatever problems or perceived shortcomings you may have, you're *a worthwhile person* who is trying to do a difficult job to the best of your abilities. You are in *"good faith."* Since you can't always count on your patients, colleagues, and supervisors to reinforce you for your efforts, you have to learn to provide your *own* reinforcement. Learn to appreciate your own skills and take pride in yourself, even when others do not communicate their appreciation.[18]

Give your accomplishments their due, even those that are relatively minor. You don't have to save a patient's life or do something dramatic to feel that you scored an achievement that day. Congratulate yourself for the deceptively simple things you do that nonetheless make a difference in someone's life. If you're a dental hygienist, for instance, every day you make people feel better about themselves by giving them a more attractive smile. If you're a medical technologist, the tests you perform each day contribute to numerous people's health by alerting physicians to various states of illness and dysfunction. And, regardless of what field you're in, you probably chat with patients during the course of each day, helping to relieve their anxieties or instructing them about how to maintain/improve their health. Just having a congenial conversation with someone is something you can feel good about at the end of your workday. Maybe you were the only single person who talked to that patient all day. To him or to her, that counted for a lot.

As much as possible, accentuate the positives of your work. You may want to write down all the *good* things that happened during the day so that you can have a written record of the positive aspects of your job to which you can refer when you have doubts about your work and yourself. Balance the frustrations and failures with the satisfactions and successes.[19] Develop the perspective of seeing the glass as half *full* rather than half empty.

When failures do occur, do not interpret the results self-referentially.[20] If you know that you did everything possible to help that patient, don't blame yourself. Universal success is not possible and you'll be chronically disappointed if you expect perfect results all the time.

Since some of the routine tasks you do can become boring and unsatisfying, try to focus on the human contact rather than the actual task. Cleaning out a tracheotomy, for example, becomes much more rewarding when you emphasize the emotional involvement and rapport. Focusing on the process, rather than on the end result, can help guard against burnout.

Set realistic goals for yourself and your work. Unrealistic goals are ultimately self-defeating, so lower your expectations. As Veninga and Spradley note, "hitching your wagon to a star can cause enormous stress if it is a million light-years beyond our galaxy."[21] Make sure your goals are attainable. You'll be better off if your goals are specific, concrete, and achievable. Instead of convincing yourself that you can "save" patients from all that ails them, remind yourself that you have a *chance* to help them in some small way. Setting specific, measurable goals will be more reinforcing for you. Rather than setting a vague goal of improving a cardiac patient's condition, establish shorter-term, concrete goals such as improving his knowledge about nutrition or talking to him about his medications.

A sense of humor can go a long way in reducing emotional strain. This doesn't mean that you shouldn't take your job seriously, but simply that you should try to see and appreciate the funny things that may occur in your job. Any viewer of the M*A*S*H television show has seen how the surgeons use humor to cope with the tremendous pressure they experienced. While still maintaining compassion for their patients and utilizing excellent technical skills, they attempted to find some light note in what was otherwise a grim situation. Negative humor (i.e., laughing *at* patients) is not appropriate and will only wind up in your feeling guilty about poking fun at people in a cruel way; but the appropriate use of humor can be beneficial for both you and your patients. Even something as seemingly silly as a kazoo band composed of staff members who march from room to room playing request numbers from patients can lift the spirits of both staff and patients alike.[22]

Visual imagery exercises brightened by a touch of humor can also be helpful in relieving tension. Using your imagination, you can visualize a comic situation that reduces some of the negative feelings you're experiencing. This can be especially constructive when you're forced to deal with someone whose manner is hostile or aggressive. One author suggests a particularly vivid image to use with irate physicians.[23] If a doctor is ranting and raving about something, you can focus on the top of his head and imagine it twirling above him like a helicopter blade to lift him right off the floor. Another humorous visual image can be that of the doctor wearing a bathing suit, or nothing at all. While you haven't changed the doctor's behavior, your imagination has insulated you from your reaction to it. You see that "the doctor has no clothes."

A strong religious faith or spiritual philosophy can also give you personal strength. Maslach[24] notes that this can give meaning to work, provide hope and inspiration, and be a source of comfort and joy. This doesn't mean that you necessarily have to be an active member of an organized religion, but it does suggest that you explore your own spiritual nature to develop fundamental guidelines for thinking and feeling. If you don't derive comfort and strength from the religion you were raised in, it could be worthwhile to investigate some other faiths or philosophies. Some people's lives have been completely turned around just by reading one book, be it the Bible, ancient Buddhist writings, or a treatise on existential philosophy.

You're more than just a job title and there should be more to your life than work. Your nonworking hours need to incorporate the *presence* of *something else* and shouldn't merely be the absence of work.[25] Strive for a full and varied private life to complement your public one. Helping others shouldn't be the only means by which you enhance your self-concept. If it becomes the single thing that makes you feel good about yourself, you may overcommit your time and energy to work.[26] You then increase your chances of becoming fatigued and thus less effective at work. A vicious cycle can develop in which you work even harder, still putting all your emotional "eggs" into one basket (work), but wind up being too tired and stressed to do anything *at* work. As your performance deteriorates, so does the satisfaction you originally obtained from work, and everything can seem to be caving in on you.

Obtain your emotional gratification from a variety of sources. Cultivate satisfying personal relationships off the job. Even when your personal interactions at work don't go well, all is not lost because you can receive emotional support and affection elsewhere. Have a broad base of activities. Learn to do lots of things well, increasing your self-esteem as you master new challenges and develop other skills besides those you utilize at work.

Develop the ability to compartmentalize your work and personal lives. Leave work at work and home at home. It's especially important to ease the transition from work to home. Maslach[27] notes the analogy of a scuba diver who will get the painful condition known as the "bends" if he returns too quickly to an environment of normal atmospheric pressure. To avoid this, the diver makes a gradual transition out of the high-pressure environment and decompresses. Health care workers who work in environments of high emotional pressure similarly need time to decompress before crossing into the normal pressure of private life. Make the most of the time between leaving work and getting home. If you commute by train or bus, you have the opportunity to read or rest on your way home. If you have to stand, observe other passengers, ads, even graffiti. Driving can be quite stressful, so try listening to relaxing music or a cassette tape on which a book is read aloud. Some people enjoy stopping off at a bar to unwind after work, but this technique is a fallacy. Alcohol is a depressant. Stopping off in a quiet environment (i.e., a park) can allow you to decompress. If distance is feasible, walking home (or part of the way) is, figuratively and literally, a change of pace.

Once home, continue to cool down. Don't talk about your job for at least an hour. Concentrate on talking about pleasant things, putting your work problems on the back burner until you can deal with them in a less intensely emotional way. Many authorities recommend slowing down physically and mentally by taking a hot bath, sitting in a sauna or Jacuzzi, getting a massage, or taking a nap. Others advise against going from too much to too little stress. Hanson[28] believes that it is preferable to switch to something *else* that is *also* stressful. Rather than just staring at the ceiling or mindlessly watching television, recharge yourself by engaging in an alternate demanding activity that, although requiring full concentration, involves different *circuits* of the brain and body. If your job is sedentary, vigorous physical activity can diminish your work stress. If you find your job boring and mentally unchallenging, read thought-provoking books or enroll in a college course.

Don't fall into the easy trap of practicing your profession after working hours. Dietitians may feel obligated to counsel their friends about their eating habits at parties and restaurants; physical therapists may find themselves performing kinesiological analyses and evaluating the body mechanics of people working out at the local gym. But by doing this, they retain their professional persona for extended lengths of time. Their 8-hour workday can become twice as long if they continue to concern themselves with aspects of their health care field. Since a full day of performing a health care job can greatly tax your emotional and physical reserves, don't compound the problem by practicing health care during your off-hours.

Be *selfish* about your leisure time. You've earned it, and you should use it as you see fit. If you want to be alone, that's your right. If you feel like socializing, then socialize. Develop hobbies and other avocational interests. Consider moonlighting in an unrelated job; in addition to the extra income, it also gives you a chance to meet new people, develop new skills, and work in an environment that's far removed from the health care setting.

Chronic stress (such as that encountered in most health care jobs) can result in physical symptoms such as weight disorders, muscle tension, increased blood sugar and cholesterol, headaches, and muscle tension. These symptoms are unpleasant at best and can even be life-threatening. To reduce the health risks, it is essential to learn how to relax, both physically and mentally. The method(s) you choose is up to you; just be sure you practice the technique(s) until you become proficient.

Transcendental meditation (TM) was a popular technique in the 1960s and 1970s. Although it has since lost some of its popularity, it remains a possible method for reducing stress. There are still schools of transcendental meditation, but you can teach yourself how to meditate. You'll need to choose one word (called a mantra) that you'll be continually repeating during your meditative period. Some people are able to use a word with a positive meaning (i.e., love and peace) while others use words with a neutral connotation (i.e., plant or sea). Strict followers of TM use an unfamiliar word without any meaning to the user so that everyday thoughts and concerns are removed. Appropriate mantras can be sounds like "um," "ah," "om," "sha-ram," or "das-car." Find a quiet spot where you won't be interrupted. Take your shoes off and sit in a comfortable chair. Be sure that you don't do your meditation on a full stomach or after you've had a lot of caffeine. Practice saying the mantra silently, softly, and then more loudly, while deeply exhaling between each repetition. Don't concern yourself with the pace or tone of your chanting; just allow it to develop.

Self-hypnosis can also be helpful for achieving relaxation. A psychologist or hypnotherapist can teach you this technique in a few sessions. You can practice it on your own by giving yourself a mental suggestion of relaxation.[29] Find a secluded place where you can sit in a chair with your feet on the floor. Close your eyes and take a few deep breaths. Tell yourself something similar to this:

As I sit here, I feel my feet growing heavy. They're getting heavier and heavier. It's a good feeling. I'm starting to feel relaxed.

Now the sensation is moving up. It's in my legs. They're growing heavy. It feels very relaxing.

My lower body is totally relaxed. I don't want to move. I couldn't move even if I wanted to because my legs are very heavy, very relaxed.

The sensation is moving up into my chest and shoulders. I'm letting go to the feeling. My body is slipping into deeper and deeper relaxation.

It's in my arms now. Nothing matters but the feeling. I feel completely relaxed.

The feeling is traveling up to the my head. My neck muscles feel very relaxed.

I can feel my entire body relaxed and loose. There's no tension left.

Visualization can be used to block out thoughts and allow relaxation to occur. Try to banish all thoughts; concentrate only on a pleasant visual image such as a calm ocean or clouds slowly drifting through a blue sky. Another possibility that can reduce unwanted active thinking is to build a wall of bricks, one brick at a time, in your mind.[30] Envision the ground on which the wall will be built, level the ground, place the first row of bricks on the ground, and build the wall brick by brick. When you see this image and aren't thinking about anything else, you can fade out the detailed image and allow a gray or black "nothingness" to be the image before your closed eyes.[31]

By learning to control your breathing, you can change your blood pressure and achieve a more relaxed state.[32] Practice deep breathing when you feel especially anxious or stressed. You can also do exercises such as altering your breathing so that you breathe in through your nose to a count of four and then breathe out through your open nose to a count of eight. The repetition of exhaling and inhaling this way can help to release tension. Since the complete breathing techniques used by yoga enthusiasts promote relaxation as well, it can be well worth your while to enroll in a yoga class.

The progressive relaxation technique utilized by behavioral therapists can be very helpful. The tension in the muscles is exaggerated by alternately tightening and squeezing them, then relaxing and letting go. Begin by wearing loose clothing and assuming a comfortable position such as sitting or lying on your back. Dimmed lights and soft relaxing music can promote the right atmosphere for relaxation. The muscles in each body part (i.e., left foot, right foot, lower legs, thighs, buttocks, abdomen, chest, shoulders, arms, hands, neck, and facial muscles) are stiffened, held in a tensed position for a count of five, and then relaxed. Concentrate on areas which seem to be especially tense. Helpful motions may include:

> making a fist
> spreading your fingers apart
> sucking in your abdomen
> pushing your abdomen out
> opening your mouth wide
> clenching your teeth
> smiling widely
> pursing your lips
> wrinkling your nose
> raising your eyebrows
> squeezing your buttocks together
> stretching your neck
> stiffening your thighs

Good sleep habits, proper nutrition, and exercise are essential for coping with stress. If your physical health isn't good, you'll feel fatigued and will be less equipped to handle emotional and physical strain. For optimal stress management, you'll need to combine practices that promote your physical health with those that improve your mental coping abilities. Learning to manage stress will take time and energy, but it's *an investment in yourself.* For your own sake, as well as of those whose lives you touch, make the commitment to do everything you can to cope with stress triumphantly.

*Chapter 7*

# MAKING A CAREER SWITCH

Even as far back as high school, I wanted to be a speech pathologist. I couldn't wait until I finished college and could actually start working as one. It seemed like the ideal career to me: a profession that would allow me to help others in a meaningful way, but without requiring years and years of school and training like medicine, and where jobs would be plentiful and the pay good.

But I became disillusioned after a few years. Jobs weren't as plentiful as I thought they would be. Although I was able to find a job as soon as I graduated, there weren't a whole lot of options when I wanted to switch jobs a couple years later. It wasn't as if I could just pick up my local paper and find a dozen ads for speech pathologists. There were job listings in professional publications, but most of the better ones would have involved a major relocation.

The money was another problem. The beginning salary wasn't too bad, but after 5 years of experience, I was still making what was basically the same salary (except that the cost-of-living increases made it slightly less each year). When I picked up a women's magazine and saw lots of women in high-paying, high-profile jobs in the business world, I began to feel badly that I was making half, or even less, of what they were earning. It made me feel inferior that my earning potential was so limited. Some of my sorority sisters from college had already gotten important promotions and now had impressive-sounding titles like "Vice-President of Marketing" or "Sales Manager." I felt envious that they had such terrific career advancement in such a short time. I knew that, even if I worked for 30 years, there wouldn't be any real opportunities for advancement. I'd always be a speech therapist with essentially the same duties and salary.

I began to burn out at work. The endless stream of stroke patients was depressing and I felt frustrated that I wasn't able to do more to help them. When the workday was over, I felt unsatisfied, like I hadn't really accomplished anything and didn't have anything to show for my efforts.

After a lot of soul-searching, I realized that there was only one solution. Speech pathology wasn't meeting my needs and there was no way that I could make it into the type of career I wanted. It was time for me to make a career switch into the business world. The prospect terrified me but it was also exciting at the same time. Convincing potential employers to hire me wasn't easy since I had no previous business experience, but eventually I landed a job in public relations. Things were rough economically for a while since I had to take a pay cut while I trained, but soon I was making more than I ever could have as a speech pathologist. I look forward to every day now; there's always a new challenge. I don't regret the years I spent in speech pathology, but I'm glad I had the guts to make the switch.

—Former speech pathologist,
Tulsa, Oklahoma

All of the preceding chapters of this book have offered suggestions on how to make the most of your career in nursing or allied health. But sometimes even the best advice can't solve certain problems. There will always be some aspects of health care jobs that can't be changed and that you find difficult to deal with. If your job is no longer meeting your needs or if the stress becomes more than you can handle, it may be time to move on to a different career.

## MAKING THE DECISION TO SWITCH CAREERS

People work for different reasons and they expect different things from their careers. Financial need is one of the most important reasons for working. Most people depend on their work to provide them with enough money to live on. People also rely on their jobs to provide them with an identity, since society defines who we are by what we do for a living. Work offers an opportunity to achieve something important and to utilize personal talents in a meaningful way.

Work doesn't always live up to people's expectations. When work no longer fulfills their needs, workers become dissatisfied. Some are forced by circumstances to remain in jobs they dislike. Others change jobs in hopes of finding better working conditions, a bigger salary, or a greater chance for advancement. A small minority decide that a basic change is in order and switch to an entirely different career field.

One of the most frequent reasons for switching fields is the desire for more money. Although the salaries for many allied health professions have steadily increased over the years, they still cannot compare to the income potential of other careers. Health care workers often find it much harder to live on their salaries than they had anticipated. As their priorities, needs, and desires change over the years, they find it necessary to earn more money to support the kind of life-style they want. They can become frustrated and envious when they see their peers in the business or professional worlds earn double or triple what health care workers make.

Money isn't the only factor that prompts health care workers to switch fields. Nursing and allied health professionals may be seeking higher status or more prestige than their present career offers. Health care workers *should* be respected for their expertise and dedication, but the unfortunate reality of our time is that they usually aren't. Society tends to save its respect and admiration for people in glamorous, high-paying careers. Workers in health fields may also want to switch to a career which provides them with more of a sense of authority and independence. In most health care jobs, workers feel they have little power to bring about change, make decisions, or direct and manage their own work as well as the work of others.

Some health care workers perceive a lack of advancement opportunities in their chosen career. There isn't the orderly progression of career steps that is found in the business world. A sales representative might get promoted to an assistant manager after a few years, then to a district manager, and later to a regional manager. He or she might eventually end up as a national sales manager or even a vice-president of the company. A radiation technologist or nurse, on the other hand, remains just that over the course of his or her career. Consequently, health professionals may feel that their career in health care is stagnant and want to change to a career that offers "upward mobility."

Sometimes the actual duties of health care jobs lose their appeal after the worker has performed them for several years. The repetition inherent in almost any job (not just jobs in health care) can lead to boredom and the worker may seek relief by switching to a drastically different kind of job. Health care workers may have developed additional talents over the years and want to switch to a career that offers them the chance to utilize these talents. For example, a nurse might have taken some creative writing courses on a part-time basis and decide that he or she would be happier in a job where these new communication skills would be used and appreciated. Some health care workers also reach the point where they want a job in which they can see tangible results of their work. Although they give their best effort each day, they may wonder what they've really accomplished. Since many patients get better very slowly or don't improve at all, it's easy for their care givers to feel that they haven't made a difference or that there's nothing to show for their efforts. They may begin to suspect that they'd prefer a job in business that would provide them with a sense of accomplishment (i.e., completed projects, increased sales, and so on). They feel that they have developed qualities that are worthy of greater scope. And not surprisingly, a significant number of health professionals find it difficult to continually cope with the stress that's inevitable in their work. They may come to the conclusion that the only viable solution is to switch careers.

If you're not happy at work and are considering a change to an entirely different field, make sure that it's not just the job that you're dissatisfied with. There's nothing wrong with changing careers, but you need to ascertain whether it's the particular job or the health care field itself that's causing your present dissatisfaction. Try to imagine the *ideal job* that's still *realistically possible* in your specific field. If you find this difficult to do, do some research into the classified advertising section of your professional journals. Eventually you should find a job that really appeals to you. There may be some reasons why you wouldn't be able to actually *get* that job (i.e., you're unable to move to that location or you don't have the experience to qualify for it), but ask yourself whether that ideal job would make you happier. Answer such questions as:

> Would this job provide me with sufficient salary and benefits?
>
> After I became acclimated to the job, would I still find it challenging? (Or would it start to bore me like my current job?)
>
> How stressful would this new job be? Would I be able to deal with the stress?
>
> Would I feel better about myself in the new job?
>
> If this new job doesn't work out, would there be any other positions available that would also be preferable to what I have now?
>
> If I was in a job I liked better, would I be more interested in and excited about my career field?
>
> If I was in my ideal job, would I be proud to be a member of this profession?

If you answered yes to the majority of the questions, it probably would be a good idea for you to continue working in your present health care field. But keep trying to find a job that would suit you better than the one you have now. Don't be rash about giving up your health career itself; you seem to have a good chance of being happy in health care if you can just discover the right job for you. If, on the other hand, you can't honestly answer yes to most of the questions, it may be best for you to start looking for a different career. Even the ideal job in your present field would not make you happy.

Put substantial time and energy into analyzing whether you need to change jobs or switch careers. All too often, people make career decisions with less concern, care, or expertise than they devote to buying clothes or planning a vacation.[1] If you eventually come to the conclusion that you want to leave the health care field, keep in mind that switching careers won't be easy. It can be done, and many health care workers have made the switch successfully, but it will take a lot of effort and psychological stamina on your part. And it's especially important to take off your rose-colored glasses. If you're convinced that life will be perfect in your new career, you'll only be disillusioned. No job or career field is without its problems. Those you face in your new field may be different the ones in health care, but they can be equally frustrating and stressful. You might even find that the problems you thought you left behind in health care exist in your new job as well.

As mentioned earlier, money is a major motivator for switching careers. But just because a career has the potential for high pay doesn't automatically mean that you would be making megabucks in your new career. You may know someone who makes a fortune in advertising or you can pick up a magazine that features highly successful advertising executives. But that doesn't mean that you'll approach that level if you went into advertising. Every career field has workers who achieve great success, *and* workers who are only marginal performers. Most fall somewhere in between these two extremes and earn salaries in the moderate range. This middle range can be more than what you're earning now as a health professional, but it may not be as much as you were led to believe is possible when you read about those at the top.

The business world also appeals to health care workers because it promises recognition and rewards based on each individual's performance. Superior health care professionals usually don't receive any special recognition or rewards for their efforts.

A physical therapist who has exceptionally good results in rehabilitating stroke patients or a nurse who provides consistently excellent patient care typically get the same annual raise as their less dedicated and less skillful colleagues. In the business world, however, successful employees can be rewarded with bonuses, commissions, and promotions. But be careful to keep this contrast in proper perspective. There are no guarantees that you'll be fairly rewarded for your efforts if you switch to a business field. Many businesspeople feel that they haven't received their fair due from their employers. Office politics and personalities can result in your being overlooked when it comes time for a bonus or promotion.

Although the business world offers more of a career ladder than the health care field, you'll need to remember that there's also an incredible amount of competition for the most desirable jobs. Your job performance can be exemplary, but so may that of several of your coworkers. Any time a promotional opportunity comes along, you'll be competing with two, five, or even more of your colleagues for that position. The top positions with the prestige, power, and financial rewards are relatively small in number; the lower and middle echelons form the foundation of a company. Not everyone can be a chief; businesses need plenty of Indians to function properly. Look at it this way; if you go into business, you'll have a *chance* (not guarantee) of mounting the career ladder.

Health care workers also leave their professions to search for work that would offer them more satisfaction. They seek challenging careers that would provide intellectual stimulation or allow them to express their creativity. But it's unrealistic to expect that any job will provide you with constant satisfaction. Jobs in every career field have their routine functions that, although monotonous, are a necessary part of the job. Most jobs are not varied enough to offer stimulation and new challenges every moment throughout the workday. If you have a great need to be creative or to expand your intellectual prowess, you might have to do this after working hours.

While health care jobs can be incredibly stressful, remember that jobs in other fields have their own stresses. There's no way to entirely avoid stress in any sector of the work world. Regardless of what field you're in, you're going to be subject to some stressful elements in your work. If you switch from health care to another field, you'll probably only wind up swapping one set of stresses for another. The business world can be very high-pressure, with deadlines, quotas, and budgets to meet. Bosses can be coldly unsympathetic and demanding, concerned only with the bottom line. Ulcers, heart disease, and hypertension, after all, are not uncommon to businesspeople!

When you can accept the fact that you'll never find a career in which everything is perfect, but you still feel that you'll be happier in a different career, you're ready to start planning for your big switch.

## Taking Action to Switch Careers

Jobs, particularly those in fields other than that which you have experience in, don't come looking for you. You have to go look for them and to develop a strategy for convincing potential employers to hire you. There *is* a demand for your talents, but it's seldom a highly visible one. You're not going to pick up the classified section of your local newspaper and see this listing:

ATTENTION, ALLIED HEALTH PERSONNEL
Looking for a career change? Fortune 500 company is looking for several health professionals to fill openings in the sales, marketing, and personnel departments. Salary is negotiable but is guaranteed to be at least 30% higher than your current salary. Excellent benefits and advancement opportunities. Reply Box 78-A.

To make a successful career switch from health care to a different field, you're going to need a great deal of creativity and initiative. You may be tempted to procrastinate rather than take direct action, but this is counterproductive. Your chances of switching careers are virtually nonexistent if you're unwilling to expend the necessary time and energy. If you can think of a hundred reasons to delay making your career switch strategy, perhaps you're not really ready to leave the health care field.

But if you're truly dissatisfied in your present career, you'll do everything you can to find a career you'll be happier in.

The first thing you've got to do is to decide which career fields interest you. Be realistic about this. Don't choose fields that require long years of schooling and training unless you're prepared to go back to school. Law might sound fascinating to you, for example, but if you're financially or psychologically unable to spend 3 years at law school, don't envision passing the bar. There is nothing frivolous about retraining for a new career, unless you're just going back to school in an effort to postpone solving your career problem. Since retraining can be costly both in time and money, you'd be better off waiting to decide about formal retraining once you are *already engaged in a new career*. If you think you'd like a career in public relations, first get an entry-level job in the PR field. Don't rush to sign up for a college degree program until you're sure you *like* your new career. Once you're fairly certain that you're happy in public relations, you can take college courses on a part-time basis. In many instances, employers will subsidize your tuition costs.

Consider going to a psychologist or career counselor for vocational aptitudes and interests tests. This can give you a good idea of the sort of job that would be right for you. Your library is another excellent source of career information. Almost any library has the reference book entitled *Dictionary of Occupational Titles*. This is a U.S. Government publication that defines and classifies over 20,000 occupations. The *D.O.T.* rates each occupation by the complexity of data, people, and things. When you have an idea of the type of job you'd like to pursue, check the classified ads of your newspaper to see what jobs are actually available in the community you'd like to live in.

Don't sit and think *too* long analyzing possible career options. No matter how much time you spend on researching potential new careers, you'll never know for sure that you'd like a particular field until you're actually working in it. There are no guarantees that you'll like your new career. All you can do is try it and see how it goes. Choose a career you're reasonably sure you'd like and then plunge into it.

Health care workers are used to helping others. It can be a jolt when the situation is reversed and they become the recipients of other people's help. Asking for and accepting assistance might not come naturally to you, but it can be essential in your job search. Accept help from anyone who offers it and don't be too proud to ask for it. Don't pass up any opportunities; you never know where a lead may take you. In your professional and personal lives, you've established hundreds of contacts with a variety of people. Enlist the help of patients, coworkers, friends, relatives, neighbors, classmates, members of church or clubs you belong to, even your doctor and dentist. Don't, however, put people on the spot by asking if they know of any job openings in the career you'd like to go into. Chances are that they really wouldn't know or be in a position to discuss any available position with you. Instead, ask them something like, "Do you know anyone in the public relations field whom I could speak to so I could get more insight into the profession?" The people you're referred to may be able to let you know about any openings in their companies, as well as rumored and actual vacancies elsewhere.

You'll also need to regularly check the classified ads of your newspaper. Keep in mind, though, that many jobs are not advertised in this section. Some vacant positions are listed with an employment agency or are filled by walk-in applicants who file applications with the personnel department. Also remember that there are many other people reading those same ads and the competition can be fierce. Don't get discouraged by this; look at it as a challenge to make your resume and your interview stand out among all the others.

Employment agencies may or may not be helpful. It depends on the employment agency and, especially, the counselor you're assigned to. If you go to an agency which is fee-paid, you won't have to pay a fee for any leads they give you. Even if you land a job, your employer (not you) will pay the fee. The disadvantage, as noted earlier, is that the agency isn't necessarily operating in *your* best interests. Keep an open mind about any positions they refer you to. It may *be* a golden opportunity that's tailored for you, or it could be a job that's available because no one can stand it. Don't let your counselor persuade you to take a job you've got all the wrong vibes about.

Spend enough time and effort on your resume to make it an effective marketing tool. A good resume is an advertisement.

To advertise effectively, you must have a well-conceived product and identify parties who would be interested in it. An effective resume means that you define your product's attributes. Since *you*'re the product, you need to spell out your skills, accomplishments, and expertise. After you do this, you can identify organizations who need this product (your services).

In a traditional resume, your current and past employment situations are listed in chronological order. Although this is still the most frequently utilized format, it is the wrong one for you. By the time the person reading the resume is finished with it, he will see you just as a nurse, therapist, or technician, not as someone who is in any way qualified to fill the position in question. You may have put a job objective at the top of your resume, i.e. "an outside sales position with a consumer products firm"; but the resume reader, unless highly imaginative, won't be able to make the connection as to how your skills could transfer to the business setting.

A *functional* resume stresses your *skills*. Pick three to six skills that are relevant to the job you're applying for. Tie these skills into the potential position, using business jargon whenever possible. Identify parallels between the skills you gained in your health care jobs and the new career you're seeking. If you're applying for a sales position, for example, don't just list your former duties as "patient care." Articulate your skills in a way that relates to the job you want, i.e., "Anticipated client's needs for medical care, rehabilitation, and discharge planning"; this relates to anticipating customer needs in preparation for a sales presentation. If you're an occupational therapist who's designed a new hand splint, list this as "PRODUCT DEVELOPMENT" and explain exactly what you did. Product development can also include designing a more effective program or technique. Other examples include:

### COST REDUCTION
As a nurse or therapist, you may have saved your employer a significant amount of money by recruiting volunteer workers, purchasing less expensive supplies, improving staff scheduling.

## ENLARGED LINE OF CURRENT PRODUCTS AND SERVICES

As a dietitian, you may have started an innovative outpatient diet program. As a physical therapist, you may have developed a well-baby infant stimulation program. Anything you did to start a new program resulted in more business and profit for your facility. This ability could be helpful in a sales or marketing position in which you could stimulate additional sales or identify new markets.

## IMPROVED COMPANY OPERATIONS

You may have contributed new procedures or developed workshops that helped your facility run more effectively. Just as you were a valuable employee in your health care job, so will you be in the business world.

## ORGANIZED TIME, MATERIALS, PERSONNEL

Every nurse has had to organize supplies, delegate responsibility, and supervise aides within some severely limited time restrictions. This is a quality that is necessary for any manager or administrator.

## HANDLED CLIENT COMPLAINTS

Any health care worker with patient contact has to deal with patient complaints. The ability to tactfully handle complaints and resolve them to both parties' mutual satisfaction would allow you to be successful in a customer service position.

### TURNING OLD SKILLS TOWARD NEW HORIZONS

The following list is not all-inclusive, but provides a springboard from which you can analyze the skills you've gained through your work in health care. As the list illustrates, there are a great many abilities that health professionals develop and utilize every day on their jobs. For example, they're naturals at marketing and sales careers since they're experienced at anticipating needs, providing information, listening, responding, and motivating. Their expertise in dealing with people can also be put to good use in personnel and management positions.

## COMMUNICATION SKILLS

*Counseling and advising* (necessary for jobs in customer services, management positions, consultant positions, personnel work, public relations)

Art/music/dance therapists
Athletic trainers
Dietitians
Nurses
Occupational therapists
Physical therapists
Physician's assistants
Psychiatric/mental health technicians
Psychologists
Public/community health educators
School health educators
Social workers
Specialists for the visually handicapped
Speech-language pathologists and audiologists
Therapeutic recreation specialists

*Explaining and instructing* (necessary for sales jobs, customer service, public relations, advertising, instructional positions)

Art/music/dance therapists
Athletic trainers
Dental hygienists
Dietitians
Educational therapists
Health sciences librarians
Nurses
Occupational therapists
Opticians
Optometric and ophthalmic assistants
Orthoptists

Physical therapists
Physician's assistants
Psychologists
Public/community health educators
Rehabilitation workers
Respiratory therapists
School health educators
Science/technical/medical writers
Social workers
Specialists for the visually handicapped
Speech-language pathologists and audiologists
Therapeutic recreation specialists

*Interviewing* (necessary for jobs in personnel, management, and journalism)

Art/music/dance therapists
Dental hygienists
Dietitians
Medical and science writers
Medical assistants
Nurses
Occupational therapists
Physical therapists
Psychiatric/mental health technicians
Psychologists
Public health/community health educators
Rehabilitation counselors
School health educators
Social workers
Speech-language pathologists
Therapeutic recreation specialists

*Mediation and conflict resolution* (necessary for jobs in public relations, customer service, sales, and other jobs with heavy public contact)

Nurses

Psychologists

Social workers

*Motivation and persuasion* (necessary for jobs in sales, advertising, public relations, fund raising, management)

Art/music/dance therapists

Athletic trainers

Dental hygienists

Dietitians

Nurses

Occupational therapists

Physical therapists

Physician's assistants

Psychiatric/mental health technicians

Psychologists

Public health/community health educators

Rehabilitation counselors

School health educators

Social workers

Speech-language pathologists and audiologists

Therapeutic recreation specialists

Vocational rehabilitation therapists

*Public relations work* (necessary in sales, advertising, public relations)

Any job in which you promote your profession or facility or program where you work

*Public speaking* (necessary for public relations and advertising, management, lecturer positions, and other business jobs)

Workers in the following fields may have spoken in front of small or large groups:

Athletic trainers

Dental hygienists

Dietitians

Medical/scientific/technical writers

Nurses

Occupational therapists

Physical therapists

Psychologists

Public health/community health educators

School health educators

Social workers

Speech-language pathologists and audiologists

*Writing* (necessary for most business jobs)

Workers in the following fields are skilled at writing clear, concise reports:

Art/dance/music therapists

Biostatisticians

Health services administrators

Nurses

Occupational health and safety professionals

Occupational therapists

Physical therapists

Psychiatric/mental health technicians

Psychologists

Public health/community health educators

School health educators

Science, medical, and technical writers

Rehabilitation counselors

Social workers

Speech-language pathologists

Therapeutic recreation specialists

## DESIGN/PLANNING SKILLS

*Creating* (of benefit to most jobs, including research development, sales, and management positions)

Art/dance/music therapists

Biomedical engineers

Dietitians

Nurses

Occupational health and safety professionals

Occupational therapists

Physical therapists

Psychologists

Public health/community health educators

Rehabilitation counselors

Social workers

Specialists for the visually handicapped

Speech-language pathologists

Therapeutic recreation specialists

*Initiating* (helpful in any job)

Any health care job in which you discovered and used new ideas and approaches

*Planning skills* (important for management positions)

Art/music/dance therapists

Biomedical engineers

Dietitians

Emergency medical technicians

Health services administrators

Nurses

Occupational therapists

Physical therapists

Physician's assistants

Psychologists

Public health/community health educators

Rehabilitation counselors

Social workers

Speech-language therapists

Therapeutic recreation specialists

### INVESTIGATIVE SKILLS

*Evaluating* (necessary for insurance adjusting, personnel, sales, management, customer service, and other business positions)

Art/dance/music therapists

Athletic trainers
Biomedical engineers
Biostatisticians
Dietitians
Emergency medical technicians
Environmentalists
Health sciences administrators
Nurses
Occupational health and safety professionals
Occupational therapists
Physical therapists
Physician's assistants
Psychologists
Public health/community health educators
Rehabilitation counselors
Social workers
Speech-language pathologists and audiologists

*Inspecting* (necessary for quality control or insurance adjusting positions)

Athletic trainers
Clinical lab services
Dental hygienists
Dental technicians
Emergency medical technicians
Nurses
Occupational therapists
Orthotists
Physical therapists
Physician's assistants
Prosthetists
Speech-language pathologists

*Investigating* (necessary for credit management, research, personnel, customer service jobs)

Art therapists

Audiologists
Biomedical engineers
Biostatisticians
Clinical laboratory services
Dance therapists
Dictitians
Environmentalists
Medical/science/technical writers
Music therapists
Nurses
Occupational health and safety professionals
Occupational therapists
Physical therapists
Physician's assistants
Psychologists
Rehabilitation counselors
Social workers

## MANAGERIAL/ADMINISTRATIVE SKILLS

*Budgeting* (necessary for management positions)
  Dietitians
  Health sciences librarians
  Health services administrators
  Nurse administrators
  Occupational therapists
  Physical therapists
*Coordinating* (necessary for outside sales, research, personnel, management positions)
  Any health care job in which you had to handle numerous events involving different people/qualities/information/activities in a logical time sequence. May include:
  Clinical laboratory personnel
  Dental assistants

Dietitians
Emergency medical technicians
Health services administrators
Medical assistants
Nurses
Occupational therapists
Opthalmic assistants and technicians
Optometric assistants and technicians
Physical therapists
Physician's assistants
Psychiatric/mental health technicians
Radiation technologists
Rehabilitation counselors
Respiratory therapists
Social workers
Speech therapists
Therapeutic recreation specialists

*Decision-making* (necessary for managerial positions)
Emergency medical technicians
Nurses
Occupational health and safety professionals
Occupational therapists
Physical therapists
Physician's assistants
Speech therapists

*Problem-solving* (necessary in sales, public relations, customer service, management, and almost any other business position)
Art/music/dance therapists
Athletic trainers
Biomedical engineers
Dietitians
Health services administrators
Nurses
Occupational health and safety professionals

Occupational therapists

Orthotists and prosthetists

Physical therapists

Physician's assistants

Psychologists

Public health/community health educators

Rehabilitation counselors

Social workers

Specialists for the visually handicapped

Speech-language pathologists

Therapeutic recreation specialists

*Recruiting* (necessary in sales, personnel, and management jobs)

Any health care job in which you attempted to acquire the services or support of other people (i.e., obtaining a family member's assistance in the patient's rehabilitation program or recruiting high-school students to work as volunteers). May include:

Health services administrators

Nurses

Occupational therapists

Physical therapists

Psychologists

Public health/community health educators

Social workers

Speech therapists

*Scheduling* (necessary in sales, personnel, and management jobs)

The following jobs may have offered opportunities to develop expertise in scheduling:

Dietitians

Health services administrators

Nurses

Occupational therapists

Pharmacists

Physical therapists
Rehabilitation counselors
Respiratory therapists
Social workers
Speech therapists

*Supervising and delegating* (necessary for all supervisory positions)

Any health care job in which you were responsible for directly overseeing or distributing the tasks and responsibilities of colleagues, assistants, aides, volunteers. May include:

Chief dietitians
Chief nuclear medicine technologists
Chief of pharmacy services
Chief radiation technologists
EEG technologists
Head respiratory therapists
Medical records administrators
Medical technologists
Nurses
Occupational therapists
Physical therapists

### Manual/Physical Skills

*Strength and stamina* (necessary for heavy labor jobs)
Athletic trainers
Dance therapists
Emergency medical technicians
Nurses
Occupational therapists
Physical therapists

*Manual dexterity* (necessary for skilled labor positions)
Art therapists
Dental assistants

Dental hygienists
Dental technicians
Medical illustrators
Nurses
Occupational therapists
Orthotists
Prosthetists
Surgical technologists
   *Using technical instruments and machines* (necessary for hi-tech jobs)
Diagnostic medical sonographers
EEG technologists and technicians
Emergency medical technicians
Nuclear medicine technologists
Nurses
Ophthalmic technicians
Optometric technicians
Physical therapists
Radiation technologists
Respiratory therapists
Surgical technologists

## NUMERICAL/INFORMATION MANAGEMENT

   *Ability to access information* (necessary in research and investigative positions)
Biomedical engineers
Biostatisticians
Health services librarians
Medical records personnel
Occupational health and safety professionals
Psychologists
Public health/community health educators

Science/technical/medical writers

Social workers

*Calculating* (necessary in statistical, clerical, and bookkeeping jobs)

Biostatisticians

Clinical laboratory workers

Dietitians

Health services administrators

Medical records personnel

Nurses

Pharmacists

*Computer skills* (important in a variety of business positions)

Any health care job in which you regularly use a computer

*Interpreting data* (necessary for statistical, marketing, sales, and other business jobs)

Biomedical engineers

Biostatisticians

Clinical laboratory workers

Dietitians

Emergency medical technicians

Environmentalists

Medical records personnel

Medical/science/technical writers

Nurses

Occupational health and safety professionals

Physical therapists

Physician's assistants

*Record keeping* (necessary for clerical, research, marketing, sales, management positions)

Animal technicians

Art/dance/music therapists

Biomedical engineers

Biostatisticians

Dental assistants

Dental hygienists
Dietitians
Health services administrators
Medical assistants
Medical records personnel
Nurses
Occupational health and safety professionals
Occupational therapists
Ophthalmic assistants and technicians
Pharmacists
Physical therapists
Physician's assistants
Psychiatric/mental health technicians
Psychologists
Radiation technologists
Rehabilitation counselors
Respiratory therapists
Social workers
Speech-language pathologists and audiologists
Therapeutic recreation specialists

## PERSONAL ATTRIBUTES

*Ability to work independently or with minimal supervision* (necessary for outside sales, management, and other business positions)
Art/dance/music therapists
Athletic trainers
Biomedical engineers
Biostatisticians
Clinical chemists
Dental hygienists
Dietitians

Emergency medical technicians
Environmentalists
Health sciences librarians
Health services administrators
Medical records administrators
Medical technologists
Microbiologists
Nurses
Occupational health and safety professionals
Occupational therapists
Orthotists and prosthetists
Pharmacists
Physical therapists
Physician's assistants
Psychologists
Public health/community health educators
Radiation technologists
Rehabilitation counselors
Respiratory therapists
School health educators
Science/medical/technical writers
Social workers
Specialists for the visually handicapped
Speech-language pathologists and audiologists

*Ability to work under pressure* (necessary for sales, journalism, management, other business positions)

Emergency medical technicians
Nurses
Respiratory therapists
Surgical technologists

Depending on the situation, other high-pressure jobs could include:

Clinical laboratory personnel
Occupational therapists

Pharmacists

Physical therapists

Physician's assistants

Radiation technologists

*Relating well to all sectors of the population* (necessary for sales, customer service, and all positions involving heavy public contact)

Art/music/dance therapists

Dental assistants

Dental hygienists

Dietitians

EEG technologists and technicians

Emergency medical technicians

Medical assistants

Nuclear medicine technologists

Nurses

Occupational therapists

Optometric and ophthalmic assistants and technicians

Physical therapists

Physician's assistants

Podiatric assistants

Psychologists

Public health/community health educators

Respiratory therapists

Social workers

Specialists for the visually handicapped

Speech-language pathologists

You'll need to choose a few skills that apply to the job you're seeking. If you're applying to several jobs in a variety of fields, you'll probably need to write a different resume for each position. Include only those skills and abilities that validate your potential to do the job you seek. Don't forget skills you've developed outside of your job, such as hobbies, clubs, and civic organizations. If you've held a leadership position in an avocational or civic club, be sure to include this since it attests to your ability to direct, organize, and manage people.

Put a job objective on your cover letter or, preferably, your resume. Be specific about this objective. Don't just say you want a sales job—state that you're seeking a job in *pharmaceutical* sales. Make sure that your job objective fits the job you're applying for. You don't want to send a resume stating that you're looking for a job in pharmaceutical sales to an insurance agency or stock brokerage firm. A good example of a job objective would be: "A public relations position involving program planning and co-ordination, and which requires an ability to work with diverse groups and develop publicity and promotional campaigns."

A resume for a nurse who wants a sales job should look something like this:

## RESUME

Name
Address
Phone number:

*Job objective:* A position in pharmaceutical sales.

*Professional skills*

> Assessment of needs  Motivating
> Data analysis  Public relations
> Problem solving  Excellent written and oral
>   communication skills
> Knowledge of pharmacology and biomedical sciences

*Professional experiences*

> Served as a fieldwork supervisor
> Presented seminars to nursing and medical personnel on burn care.
> Designed and implemented a training program for student nurses.

Convinced administrators to utilize a more effective solution during debriding procedures.

Organized a study group for nurses in burn units.

*Education*

M.S.N., 1978, Medical University of the U.S.A., New York, NY

B.S.N., 1972, Liberal Arts College, College Town, New Jersey

*Employment*

1981 to present: Metropolis Hospital, Metropolitan, New York
Head nurse, Burn Unit.
Duties included supervision of thirty nursing and other personnel.

1978 to 1981: Any Medical Center, Any Town, New Jersey
Staff nurse, Intensive care unit.

1972 to 1976: Community Hospital, Suburbia, New Jersey
Staff nurse, Medical and surgical floor.

A resume for an occupational therapist who is seeking a job in employee training might read:

## RESUME

Name
Address
Phone number

*Job objective:* An entry-level position in employee training.

*Professional skills*

| | |
|---|---|
| Instructing | Superior oral and written |
| Motivating | communication skills |

Needs assessment                    Excellent interpersonal
Program development                   skills

*Professional experiences*

Developed a program to train mentally retarded and psychiatric clients in daily living skills.

Presented workshops to mental health personnel on a variety of subjects.

Performed in-depth evaluations to assess clients' needs.

Coordinated an interdisciplinary program in stress management.

Supervised student therapists.

*Education*

Bachelor of Science in Occupational Therapy, Summa Cum Laude, 1980, Some College, Little Rock, Arkansas

Additional courses during this past year in adult education, business writing, psychology, and business.

*Employment*

1983 to present: Memorial Hospital, South City, Virginia
Title: Mental health therapist.
Duties: Responsible for evaluation and treatment of a caseload of 60 clients.

1980 to 1983: Urban Psychiatric Center, New Orleans, Louisiana
Title: Occupational therapist.
Duties: Directed therapeutic program on a 30-bed unit.

*Additional experiences*

Member of Toastmaster's Club for development of public speaking skills.

Editor of civic club newsletter.

Your resume should be one to two pages. It's permissible to send a Xeroxed copy of your typed cover letter. This letter should consist of a few paragraphs that state the position you're interested in, and why, that your resume is enclosed, and that you're looking forward to discussing your qualifications during a personal interview. Try a cover letter like this:

Address

Date

Title of person you're sending the resume to
Company
Address

Dear Mr. _____ or Ms. _____:
      or
Dear Sir or Madam (if you don't know the name of the person):

As you see from the enclosed resume, I have eight years of successful experience as a dietitian: the past three in a supervisory position. During this time, I've developed a keen interest in the business world. I now feel that a management position in business would be more challenging and offer more opportunity for growth than my current field. I seek a position in which effective work results in tangible recognition. Your management trainee position advertised in the *Local News* strikes me as that kind of opportunity.

While I may not have directly applicable experience, I am a quick learner who always presents herself in a professional manner. My years of experience in the health field attest to my interpersonal skills. I'm organized, energetic, and dedicated to excellence in every project I undertake.

My salary requirements are negotiable. I am willing to begin at a lower salary than I currently earn in order to change career fields.

I look forward to the opportunity to interview with your company.

Sincerely,

Your name

When you land an interview, always be enthusiastic, positive, and self-confident. Too many health care workers feel apologetic or ashamed about "giving up" on the career they've trained for. Avoid this type of negative thinking. You have *nothing to apologize for* or to feel badly about. Health care is a high burn-out field and it is not uncommon for health professionals to seek other jobs after working in the field for a number of years. In fact, workers in almost every field are apt to change careers at least once during their working years. This can be a healthy, growth-promoting experience, as has become widely recognized; it's certainly no reason to feel you failed. Rather, you show courage. You made the choice to become a health care worker in the past. At the time, it appeared that a health career would meet your needs. Since then, you have matured and your goals, needs, wants, and ambitions have changed.

Don't think of yourself as "just a health care worker" when you interview. You may not have a degree or experience in business, but you shouldn't feel inadequate because of this. You've developed essential skills in areas that could be applied to the business world. You've demonstrated that you have the ability to work under pressure, deal with a variety of people, and solve problems, whereas a recent college graduate in business has not. The fact that you went into nursing or allied health does not mean that you are less intelligent or less competent than people in more prestigious, higher-paying fields. The reason you are now in the health care field is that *you chose it, based on your interests at the time*. No one came to you during high school and college and told you not to go for an M.B.A. or into law or medicine because you didn't have what it takes to handle it. Health care was your own authentic choice once upon a time; but now it's your perogative to change your mind, along with all the other intervening changes, and make a different choice, one just as authentic.

After each interview, write a thank-you letter to the interviewer. It should say something like:

> Thank you for interrupting your busy schedule on Thursday, May 4th, and granting me an interview. From our discussion, I feel that my ability to motivate people, combined with my scientific knowledge, is an excellent preparation for a medical sales career. I am extremely interested in your company due to your unique product line and management philosophy.

Also report back to and thank anyone who gave you a lead, even if nothing comes of that particular one.

There will always be some anxious moments when you change careers. You're not going to get every job you apply for, and it can be hard not to take this personally. You'll need to keep reminding yourself that it's a "job fit" rejection rather than a personal rejection. Someone else fit the jobs specifications more closely than you did. But don't get discouraged. It's not easy to switch to an entirely new career field, but it *can* be done. The proof is that you probably have a few former colleagues who have successfully switched from allied health to something else. It's best if you can conduct your job search while you're still employed. You'll feel more positive about yourself and you won't be so desperate for money that you would grab at just any job.

Be flexible about your salary and level of responsibility in a new career. It calls for rebudgeting to take a pay cut or to start at the bottom, but you're trying to learn a whole new field. If you're offered a job with less pay or a less impressive title than you'd like, try to swallow your pride and take advantage of the opportunity to enter a different career. Look at it this way: When you were in school, training for your health career, no one paid you for your time and effort. In fact, you had to pay for the privilege of learning your health field. Now someone's offering to pay you to learn a new career. If that pay is somewhat lower than you've been earning, keep in mind that there's probably a very good chance that your salary will increase significantly once you gain experience. After a few years, your salary may well be double or triple what you'd be making had you stayed in health care.

As difficult as it can be, a career switch can be one of the best things you've ever done for yourself. Your career choice always matters deeply, whether it's the original choice or the second time around. And a mid-career decision to make a change doesn't *vitiate* the first choice. It was what you wanted *then*. You couldn't "throw away all that education and all those years of experience" even if you tried. They are part of you and of whatever else you do, and as such you will always be glad of them.

# REFERENCES

## CHAPTER 5. THE LATER YEARS.

1. Nudel, A. *For the woman over 50*. New York: Taplinger, 1978.

## CHAPTER 6. STRESS AND BURNOUT.

1. Muldary, T. W. *Burnout and health professionals: Manifestation and management*. Norwalk, Conn.: Appleton-Century-Crofts, 1983, p. 2.
2. Ibid, p. 89.
3. Ibid, p. 92.
4. Aiken, L. H. *Nursing in the 1980's: Crises, opportunities, challenges*. Philadelphia: Lippincott, 1982.
5. Muldary, p. 85.
6. Maslach, C. *Burnout—The cost of caring*. Englewood Cliffs, N.J.: Prentice-Hall, 1982, pp. 59–60.
7. Ibid.
8. Jacobson, S. F. Nurses' stress in intensive and nonintensive care

units. In S. F. Jacobson & H. M. McGrath (Eds.), *Nurses under stress.* New York: Wiley, 1983, pp. 61–83.

9.  Veninga, R. L., & Spradley, J. P. *The work/stress connection.* Boston: Little, Brown, 1981.
10. Edelwich, J., & Brodsky, A. *Burnout: Stages of disillusionment in the helping professions.* New York: Human Sciences Press, 1980, p. 39.
11. Muldary, p. 6.
12. Veninga & Spradley.
13. Maslach, p. 59.
14. Maslach, p. 71.
15. Maslach, p. 32.
16. Maslach, p. 72.
17. Anderson, E. R. Stress and the nursing student. In S. F. Jacobson & H. M. McGrath (Eds.), *Nurses under stress.* New York: Wiley, 1983, pp. 295–316.
18. Muldary, p. 143.
19. Maslach, p. 95.
20. Edelwich, & Brodsky, p. 212.
21. Veninga, & Spradley, p. 96.
22. Koocher, G. P. Adjustment and coping strategies among the caretakers of cancer patients. *Social Work in Health Care,* 1979, *5*(2), 145–150.
23. Donnelly, G. F. Doctoring reality—To nurse your nerves back to health. *RN,* 1979, *42*(4), 31–33.
24. Maslach, p. 106.
25. Maslach, p. 104.
26. Hall, R. C. W., Gardner, E. R., Perl, M., Stickney, S., & Pfefferbaum, B. The professional burnout syndrome. *Psychiatric Opinion,* 1979, *16*(4), 12–17.
27. Maslach, p. 102.
28. Hanson, P. G. *The joy of stress.* Kansas City: Andrews, McNeel, & Parker, 1983.
29. Gill, J. L. *Personalized stress management.* San Jose: Counseling and Consulting Services, 1983.
30. Welch, I. D., Medeiros, D. C., & Tate, G. A. *Beyond burnout.* Englewood Cliffs, N.J.: Prentice-Hall, 1982, p. 265.
31. Maslach, p. 154.
32. Schwartz, J. *Letting go of stress.* New York: Pinnacle, 1982.

## Chapter 7. Making A Career Switch.

1.  Goodman, L. H. *Alternative careers for teachers, librarians, and counselors.* New York: Monarch, 1982.

# BIBLIOGRAPHY

## Chapter 1. Deciding on a Health Career.

*Dictionary of occupational titles.* Washington, D.C.: U.S. Department of Labor, 1977.

Hopke, W. E. (Ed.). *The encyclopedia of careers and vocational guidance.* Chicago: J. G. Ferguson, 1984.

Ilk, C. R. *Student's career guide to a future in the allied health professions.* New York: Arco, 1982.

Nassif, J. Z. *Handbook of health careers.* New York: Human Sciences, 1980.

Zimmerman, B., & Smith, D. B. *Careers in health.* Boston: Beacon, 1978.

## Chapter 2. The Student Years.

Anderson, E. R. Stress and the nursing student. In S. F. Jacobson & H. M. McGrath (Eds.), *Nurses under stress.* New York: Wiley, 1983, pp. 295–316.

Kramer, M. *Reality shock.* St. Louis: Mosby, 1974.

## Chapter 3. The First Year(s).

Berliner, D. *Want a job? Get some experience. Want experience? Get a job.* New York: Amacom, 1978.

Catalyst, Inc. *Making the most of your first job.* New York: Putnam, 1981.

Elsman, M. *How to get your first job.* New York: Crown, 1985.

Moldafsky, A. *Welcome to the real world: A guide to making your first personal, financial, and career decisions.* Garden City, N.Y.: Doubleday, 1979.

Schmidt, P. J. *Making it on your first job: When you're young, inexperienced, and ambitious.* New York: Avon, 1981.

Shingleton, J. D., & Bao, R. *College to career: Finding yourself in the job market.* New York: McGraw-Hill, 1977.


## Chapter 4. The Middle Years.

Van Hoose, W. H. *Midlife myths and realities.* Atlanta: Humanics, 1985.


## Chapter 5. The Later Years.

Rogers, D. *The adult years.* Englewood Cliffs, N.J.: Prentice-Hall, 1979.

Uris, A. *Over 50.* Radnor, Penn.: Chilton, 1979.


## Chapter 6. Stress and Burnout.

Kovecses, J. S. Burnout doesn't have to happen. *Nursing 80,* 1980, *10*(10), 105–111.

McLean, A. A. *Work stress.* Reading, Mass.: Addison-Wesley, 1979.

Shubin, S. Burnout: the professional hazard you face in nursing. *Nursing 78,* 1978, *8*(7), 22–27.


## Chapter 7. Making a Career Switch.

Anderson, N. *Work with passion: How to do what you love for a living.* New York: Carroll & Graf, 1984.

Baker, N. C. *Act II*. New York: Vanguard, 1980.

Beard, M. L., & McGahey, M. J.: *Alternative careers for teachers*. New York: Arco, 1985.

Biegeleisen, J. I. *Job resumes*. New York: Grosset & Dunlap, 1976.

Bolles, R. N. *The three boxes of life*. Berkeley: Ten Speed, 1978.

Bolles, R. N. *What color is your parachute?* Berkeley: Ten Speed, 1987.

Bolles, R. N., & Crystal, J. C. *Where do I go from here with my life?* New York: Seabury, 1978.

Greco, B. *New careers for teachers*. Chicago: Dow-Jones-Irwin, 1976.

Haldane, B. *Career satisfaction and success: A guide to job freedom*. New York: Amacom, 1974.

Hoffman, V. R. *New directions for the professional nurse*. New York: Arco, 1984.

Jones, R. *The big switch*. New York: McGraw-Hill, 1980.

# INDEX

## Date Due

| MR 6 '96 | | |
|---|---|---|
| JY 28 '97 | | |
| | | |
| | | |
| | | |
| | | |
| | | |
| | | |
| | | |
| | | |
| | | |
| | | |
| | | |
| | | |
| | | |
| | | |